Subfertility

Subfertility
Recent Advances in Management and Prevention

Edited by

Rehana Rehman, MBBS, M.Phil., Ph.D., FHEA
Associate Professor, Department of Biological & Biomedical
Sciences, Aga Khan University, Karachi, Pakistan

Aisha Sheikh, MBBS, FCPS, FACE
Lecturer & Consultant Endocrinologist,
The Aga Khan University Hospital, Karachi, Pakistan

ELSEVIER

Elsevier
Radarweg 29, PO Box 211, 1000 AE Amsterdam, Netherlands
The Boulevard, Langford Lane, Kidlington, Oxford OX5 1GB, United Kingdom
50 Hampshire Street, 5th Floor, Cambridge, MA 02139, United States

Library of Congress Cataloging-in-Publication Data
A catalog record for this book is available from the Library of Congress

British Library Cataloguing-in-Publication Data
A catalogue record for this book is available from the British Library

ISBN: 978-0-323-75945-8

For information on all Elsevier publications
visit our website at https://www.elsevier.com/books-and-journals

Publisher: Dolores Meloni
Acquisitions Editor: Nancy Duffy
Editorial Project Manager: Mona Zahir
Production Project Manager: Niranjan Bhaskaran
Cover Designer: Matthew Limbert

Typeset by SPi Global, India

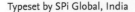

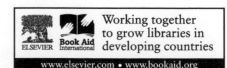

Contents

CHAPTER 3   Reproductive cycle **65**

Rabiya Ali and Rehana Rehman

CHAPTER 4   Ovarian reserve **77**

Zareen Kiran

About the editors

Dr Aisha Sheikh is MBBS, FCPS, FACE (USA), Fellowship Diabetes, Endocrinology & Metabolism (AKUH), PG Diploma in Diabetes (UK) and PG Diploma in endocrinology (UK). She is Consultant Endocrinologist and faculty member at the Aga Khan University Hospital (AKUH) and MIDEM, Karachi, Pakistan. She is a tutor for postgraduate diploma in diabetes and endocrinology at the University of South Wales (UK).

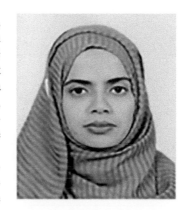

Dr Sheikh is actively involved in medical education and research and has published several research papers and book chapters and has a Google scholar citation of more than 220. She is a reviewer for several medical journals. She is an executive member and joint secretary of Pakistan Endocrine Society (PES) and member of American Association of Clinical Endocrinologists (AACE). Dr Sheikh has a keen interest in antenatal diabetes and endocrinology and has played a key role in the development of gestational diabetes mellitus guidance from the platform of South Asian Federation of Endocrine Societies (SAFES).

Dr Rehana Rehman, MBBS, MPhil, PhD, is working as Associate Professor of Physiology and Vice Chair Research & Graduate Studies in the Department of Biological and Biomedical Sciences, Aga Khan University, Karachi, Pakistan. She has been involved in teaching physiology for the past 18 years in different medical colleges. She is a well-recognized authority in the field of reproductive physiology. Her research is focused on infertility, intracytoplasmic sperm injection, physiological, and clinical and biochemical variables that facilitate implantation of embryos and maternal and fetal well-being.

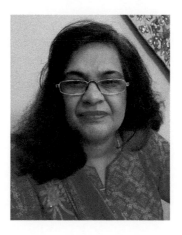

She has more than 200 publications in high-impact national and international journals and a good number of abstract presentations (oral and poster) in national and international conferences. Organizing and conducting workshops, competence-based trainings, and courses are proof of her proficiency. Her book *Five Minutes to Wellness* is based on the holistic review of all dimensions of wellness of medical students. She is an editor and author of the book *Research till Publication in Health Care* which is aimed to motivating young researchers to endorse and promote a culture of Biomedical research.

Author biographies

Dr Ahmed Mettawi is MBBCh (Cairo University), MSc (USW), holder of MRCP (UK) specialty certificate in endocrinology and diabetes, associate member of the Endocrine Society, and junior member of the ESPEN society. He is currently working as a clinical nutritionist and is deeply interested in clinical nutrition and its applications in various diseases, especially those of lifestyle etiology. Dr Mettawi holds two postgraduate diplomas in different clinical nutrition domains and is currently pursuing the American board certification in the discipline of new lifestyle medicine. He is very passionate about endocrinology topics such as resistant obesity, reproductive endocrinology, osteo-

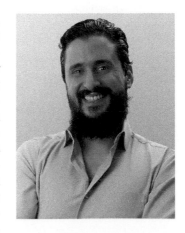

porosis, diabetic foot, and the efficacy of lifestyle interventions in managing each. Dr Mettawi's MSc dissertation focused on developing guidelines for managing and researching male osteoporosis in Egypt and a large portion of it has been published recently in the Archives of Osteoporosis Journal. He aspires to achieve the highest reproductive and metabolic health and to guide his patients down this path.

Dr Bhagwan Das, MBBS, FCPS (Pak), Fellowship Diabetes, Endocrinology & Metabolism (AKUH), is graduated from the Liaquat University of Medical and Health Sciences in 2010 with a gold medal. He did his FCPS in internal medicine from the College of Physicians and Surgeons Pakistan in 2017 and completed his fellowship in diabetes, endocrinology and metabolism from Aga Khan University Hospital, Karachi, in 2019. During his fellowship, he presented several posters at national and international endocrine conferences and published original articles, letter to the editors, and book chapters.

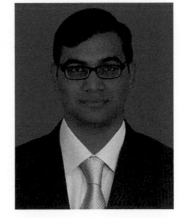

Currently, he is working as a consultant physician and endocrinologist at Cancer Foundation Hospital, Karachi. He has a special interest in reproductive endocrinology, endocrine oncology, and diabetes mellitus.

Dr Faiza Alam, MBBS, MPhil, PhD, is currently working as Assistant Professor at Pengiran Anak Puteri Rashidah Sa'adatul Bolkiah Institute of Health Sciences, Brunei, and previously worked in Aga Khan University from 2014 to 2017. After completing her master's in physiology, her research as a research scholar was dedicated toward identifying the polymorphisms of *SIRT1* gene affecting oxidative environment and fertility. It served as a logical stepping stone for studying the mechanism of action of Metformin in culture ovarian granulosa cell isolates. Broadly, her research is aimed at the causative factors of noncommunicable diseases, including obesity and diabetes and their effects on fertility.

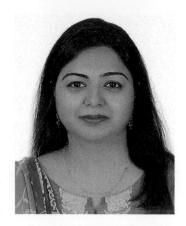

Dr Alam is also involved in educating undergraduate students about ethical principles of research, manuscript, synopsis, and thesis writing as a coordinator of the course in scientific writing and research methodology. Furthermore, she actively participated in a research grant on peer-assisted learning, in order to nurture leadership attributes and promote a more acceptable learning atmosphere.

Dr Nadeem F. Zuberi is working as Associate Professor of obstetrics and gynaecology at Aga Khan University, Karachi, Pakistan. He is an obstetrician and gynecologist/epidemiologist with over 20 years of professional practice in clinical and health research in maternal and child health. He has worked in various administrative capacities in the department of obstetrics and gynecology. These range from strengthening and uplifting undergraduate and postgraduate training programs. He has expertise and experience in planning, designing, and conducting clinical trials in community and hospital settings. His other expertise lies in performing minimal access laparoscopic gynecological surgery

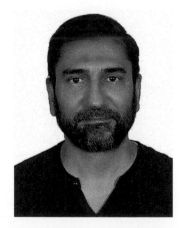

especially for severe endometriosis, women health research, and medical education. His research contribution is in various areas of women health including endometriosis, postpartum hemorrhage, preeclampsia, assisted reproduction, perinatal infections, gynecological diseases in low-income countries, clinical governance, and clinical audit.

Dr Ishrat Khan, CCT, FRCP (UK), MRCP Endocrinology (UK) and MSc (UK), is currently working as a consultant in diabetes and endocrinology (D&E) at Ysbyty Ystrad Fawr Hospital, Wales. She is an honorary lecturer for Diploma in Diabetes, Endocrinology and Acute Medicine at Cardiff University and the University of South Wales. She is a member of Wales Deanery for specialty training, responsible for supervising specialty registrars in diabetes and endocrine. She is a co-founder of the SCE Exam course for Wales, which is held annually. She has been an abstract reviewer for the Endocrine Society, USA, since 2015. She has published several articles on different subjects 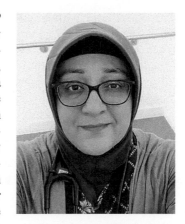 related to diabetes and endocrine. She is a faculty member of the popular Cardiff Paces course involved in teaching candidates for MRCP Paces.

Dr Rabiya Ali is an MBBS, MPhil, PhD (cont.) scholar, University of Karachi, Karachi, Pakistan. Currently she is working as Assistant Professor in the Department of Physiology at the Karachi Institute of Medical Sciences (KIMS), Karachi, Pakistan. She has been teaching physiology for the past 11 years. Her scientific research (MPhil/PhD) is based on cytokine receptor polymorphism as a root cause of implantation failure in unexplained infertility and its association with ovarian steroids and cytokines. Her work may pave the way for future research to improve pregnancy outcomes, and her approach to improving implantation by treatment with endometrial stem cells and gene therapy 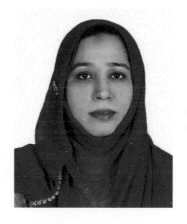 may help achieve successful implantation of blastocysts and successful outcomes of conception. She has 26 publications with Google Scholar citations with good impact factor in national and international journals. She is an active reviewer and has presented her scientific contribution in various conferences.

Dr Sairabanu Mohamed Rashid Sokwala is qualified as MBBS, MMed Internal Medicine (University of Nairobi, Kenya), PG Diploma in Diabetes, and PG Diploma in Endocrinology (University of South Wales, UK). She is pursuing an MSc in Endocrinology from the University of South Wales currently. She is a board-certified consultant physician and endocrinologist, currently working as the head of department of a multidisciplinary diabetes care center at the MP Shah Hospital, Nairobi. She has a keen interest in sleep disorders and their link with endocrine disorders. Her MMed thesis entitled "Quality of Sleep and 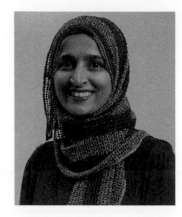 Risk for Obstructive Sleep Apnea in Ambulant Individuals with Type 2 Diabetes Mellitus at a Tertiary Referral Hospital in Kenya" was published in 2017 and has six citations to date. She is an executive member of the Kenya Diabetes Study Group, Kenya Association of Physicians, Pakistan Association of Physicians, and Diabetes Kenya. She actively delivers diabetes education through various media platforms.

Dr Sobia Sabir Ali, MBBS, FCPS, MRCP (UK), FRCP (Edin), MHPE (AKU), is Assistant Professor and Divisional Head of Diabetes & Endocrinology Services at Medical Teaching Institution, Lady Reading Hospital, Peshawar. She has the distinction of pioneering Diabetes and Endocrinology Clinical Services at Lady Reading Hospital, Peshawar. She served as Associate Dean Undergraduate Medical Education and Deputy Director, Medical Education at PGMI, Hayatabad Medical Complex. She is a supervisor and examiner for the fellowship program in endocrinology (FCPS) at the College of Physicians and Surgeons in Pakistan. Her re- 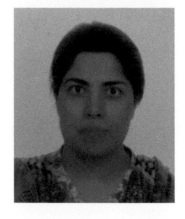 search work has been published in peer-reviewed journals, and she has been associated with various national guidelines and consensus statement forums. Dr Ali is a lifetime executive member of the Pakistan Endocrine Society, European Congress of Endocrinology, British Endocrine Society, American Association of Clinical Endocrinologists, and Endocrine Society. She has been an invited speaker at various scientific conferences. She is a faculty and program educator of the ASCEND (Academy for Science and Continuing Education in Diabetes and Obesity) program of the International Medical Press for Pakistan.

Dr Sofia Amjad holds MBBS and MPhil degrees and is currently doing PhD at Ziauddin University where she also works as Professor in the Department of Physiology. Her research is focused on the physiological, biochemical, and clinical aspect of male infertility and treatment of infertility. She has supervised/co-supervised MPhil students at Ziauddin University in reproductive physiology. Previously she also worked as Director of the Postgraduate Program at Ziauddin University and managed all postgraduate affairs from recruitment to thesis defense and mentoring of MPhil candidates in their research activities and thesis formulation. So far, she has 13 publications with more than 20 citations in Google Scholar.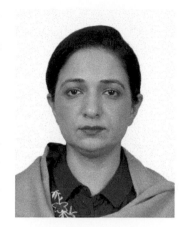

○ Lead the team of lecturers for all related activities for the entire 1 year.
○ Manage all administrative and curricular activities independently.
○ Design curriculum, strategies, and assessment plans.
○ Conduct and manage all undergraduate examination activities.

Dr Zareen Kiran, MBBS, FCPS (Medicine), MRCP (UK), FCPS (Endocrinology), is working as Assistant Professor of Endocrinology in the National Institute of Diabetes and Endocrinology, Dow University of Health Sciences, and as Consultant Endocrinologist in Aga Khan University Hospital. She teaches diabetes and endocrine topics for undergraduate students. She is one of the two members of the committee of Endocrine Module curriculum for the undergraduate MBBS program. She is also the program/curriculum team member and supervisor of Master's in Diabetes and Endocrinology in her institute, which is a recognized 2-year postgraduate course. She supervises/co-supervises MPhil and 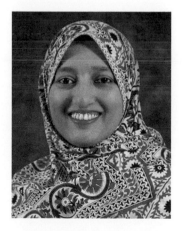 master's students in diabetes and endocrinology. She has been registered as a supervisor for fellowship training in endocrinology by the College of Physicians and Surgeons of Pakistan. Her area of interest mostly involves female endocrinology, which varied from amenorrhea to thyroid disorders in pregnancy.

Anatomy and embryology of male and female reproductive systems

1

Ahmed Sayed Mettawi

Clinical Nutrition Service, 6th of October University Hospital, 6th of October City, Giza, Egypt

Chapter outline

Subfertility. https://doi.org/10.1016/B978-0-323-75945-8.00001-3

Embryology of the male and female reproductive systems

Embryonic sexual differentiation is a very delicate process (Fig. 1.1) that starts with the genotypic determination at the time of fertilization (i.e., XY or XX) and then concludes in a manner that depends on how the gametes influence the phenotype (i.e., culminating in final pubertal and brain development events).[1] It is worth noting that most information—especially information pertaining to genetics—have been derived from mouse models since studies on human tissues are few in number and also since it has been pointed out that the developmental stages and global gene expression of both species are comparable [i.e., few exceptions exist like how *SOX2* (sex-determining region Y-box 2) and *SOX17* are two different transcription factors utilized by the primordial germ cells (PGCs) of the mouse and human species, respectively].[2,3] Sex determination has long been thought to have a predetermined default path toward a final female phenotype in the absence of the influence of the male pathway steering factors; however, recent data indicate that not only does the alternative sex development pathway need continuous active repression during the embryonic life but also that it might need to remain actively repressed for life.[4,5] Table 1.1 outlines the possible genetic errors that can disrupt such a delicate process at different stages.

Germ cell specification

Three weeks after fertilization, from the proximal epiblast-derived mesodermal portion located near the extraembryonic endoderm—at the posterior part of the primitive streak—arises a group of cells (i.e., at least six in number)[6] that display unique qualities from their surrounding tissues (i.e., larger size, clearer cytoplasm, and fewer organelles) and will later carry on their role as the PGCs.[7,8] This process has been termed "specification" and is influenced by a number of factors—that belong to the transforming growth factor-β (*TGF-β*) superfamily—produced by extraembryonic ectoderm although the cascade response of the cells depends on the expression of other factors like the wingless-type MMTV integration site member 3 (*WNT3*) (i.e., in this case to specifically respond to the bone morphogenetic proteins (*BMP*) of the TGF-β family). Genes like PR-domain containing-1 (i.e., *Prdm1* or *Blimp1* as previously called), *Prdm14*, and transcription factor AP-2 gamma (*Tfap2c*) are downstream activation targets that should be properly expressed for a successful specification to take place since—for example—*Prdm1* prevents the expression of genes that can pull the germ cell toward the somatic cell-line development.[6,9] Rodriguez and colleagues provide an excellent discussion of growth factor and genes related to sex differentiation and development that can be found in their published work.[10]

Germ cell migration and the concurrent genital ridge development
(Fig. 1.2)

For the next 1–2 weeks post specification, PGCs acquire changes in their morphology (i.e., pseudopodia) in order to carry out active amoeboid movement and successfully migrate to the hindgut and then to the genital ridge (i.e., and into the developing sex cords).[11]

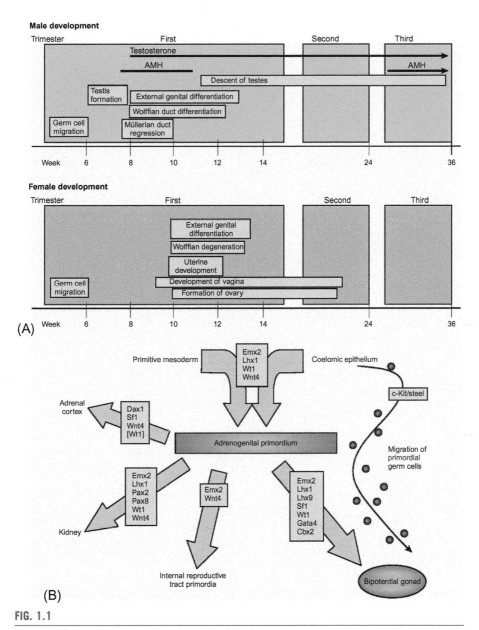

FIG. 1.1

Sexual differentiation timetable and the genetic determinants needed for the development of primordial gonads and tracts. Sexual differentiation timetable (A) and the genetic determinants needed for the development of primordial gonads and tracts (B). *Dax1*, dosage-sensitive sex reversal, adrenal hypoplasia critical region, on chromosome X, gene 1; *Emx2*, empty spiracles homeobox 2; *Gata4*, GATA-binding protein 4; *Lhx1 or 9*, homeobox protein Lim-1 or 9; *Pax2 or 8*, paired box 2 or 8; *Sf1*, steroidogenic factor-1; *Wnt4*, wingless-type MMTV integration site member 4; *Wt1*, Wilms' tumor 1.

Reproduced with permission from Arboleda VA, Quigley CA, Vilain E. Chapter 118—Genetic basis of gonadal and genital development. In: Jameson JL, De Groot LJ, de Kretser DM, et al., eds. Endocrinology: Adult and Pediatric. 7th ed. Philadelphia: Elsevier Saunders; 2016:2051–2085.e7 [Figure 118-6].

Table 1.1 Genetic factors with possible roles in sexual determination or differentiation.

Gene name or pseudonyms	Human gene locus	Protein name	Protein type	Genetic or cellular targets of factors	Action of factors	Effects of overexpression or underexpression of gene
Factors involved in both ovary and testis sex determinations						
SF1* NR5A1 FTZF1 Ad4BP	9q33	SF1	Orphan nuclear receptor/ zinc finger transcription factor	WT1, SRY, SOX9, DAX1, GNRHR, LHβ, ACTHR, AMH, AMHR, STAR, CYP11A1, CYP21A2, CYP11B1, OXT, and others	Activates transcription of many genes in the development of gonads, adrenal glands; regulates steroidogenesis; synergizes with WT1; antagonizes; DAXi. Dose-dependent activity.	KO mice (XX and XY): no gonads or adrenals; retained Müllerian structures; abnormal hypothalamus. Haploinsufficient mice: reduced but not absent adrenal function Homozygous human mutation: 46,XY sex reversal and adrenal hypoplasia Heterozygous human mutation: 46,XX normal ovary, partial adrenal insufficiency
WT1*	11p13	WT1	Zinc finger transcription factor; tumor repressor	DAX1, AMH, SRY, IGF2I, IGF1R, PDGFA, PAX2	Represses transcription; activates transcription of SRY; dose-dependent effects	XY homozygous deletion of WT1+KTS isoform: male-to-female sex reversal; XY homozygous deletion of WT1+KTS isoform: streak gonads in XX and XY. Human Denys–Drash syndrome: gonadal dysgenesis, congenital nephropathy, Wilms' tumor

Gene	Locus	Protein type	Targets	Function	Phenotype / Mutations
GATA4*	8p23.1-p22	GATA4	Zinc finger transcription factor	"GATA" DNA motif; AMH; genes encoding steroidogenic enzymes	Expressec early in both ovary and testis; interacts with FOG2	KO mice: embryonic lethal, no gonadal phenotype reported. Most human mutations cause isolated cardiac defects. Rare cases are reported with both cardiac defects and 46,XY gonadal dysgenesis
CBX2*	17q25.3	CBX2	Transcription repressor	Possibly SRY	Mediates changes in chromatin structure	KO mice (XX or XY) have retarded development of gonadal ridges; XY mice have male-to-female sex reversal. Compound heterozygous mutations cause 46,XY gonadal dysgenesis

Factors involved in testis sex determination

| SRY* | Yp11.3 | SRY | HMG-box-containing transcription factor | SF1, SOX9, CYP19A1, AMH | Bends DNA; may antagonize SOX3 | XX mice expressing transgenic Sry, female-to-male sex reversal. Human SRY mutations: 46,XY sex reversal, gonadal dysgenesis Translocation of SRY to X chromosome: 46,XX female-to-male sex reversal or ovotesticular disorder of sex development |

Continued

Table 1.1 Genetic factors with possible roles in sexual determination or differentiation—cont'd

Gene name or pseudonyms	Human gene locus	Protein name	Protein type	Genetic or cellular targets of factors	Action of factors	Effects of overexpression or underexpression of gene
SOX9*	17q24–q25	SOX9	HMG-box-containing transcription factor of SRY family	Supporting cells of gonadal primordium; WNT4, FGF9	Simulates differentiation of Sertoli cells; dosage-sensitive effects	Odsex mice: derepression of Sox9 expression in XX gonads→testis development; Human mutation: 46,XY sex reversal; gene duplication or deletion in coding and/or noncoding regions results in 46,XX or 46,XY DSD
ATRX* XH2	Xq13.1–q21.1	ATRX	Helicase; transcription factor	Widespread expression early in mouse embryogenesis, more restricted expression later	Gene regulation at interphase and chromosomal segregation at mitosis	Human mutations: α-thalassemia, mental retardation, genital anomalies→male-to-female sex reversal in 46,XY
DHH*	12q13.1	DHH	Signaling molecule	Expressed only in testis	Involved in interactions between Sertoli cells and germ cells. May regulate mitosis and meiosis in male germ cells	Strain-specific effects: XY null mice have defective Leydig cell development and are feminized. Human mutations cause 46,XY gonadal dysgenesis with peripheral neuropathy
FGF9	13q11–q12	FGF9	Growth factor	SOX9	Promotes Sertoli cell differentiation and germ cell survival	KO mice: XY sex reversal

LHCGR*	2p21	LH/CG receptor	G-protein-coupled, seven-transmembrane-peptide hormone receptor	Not applicable	Transduces LH signal to activate $G_{s\alpha}$ → cAMP. Required for Leydig cell testosterone production	Human mutation: Leydig cell hypoplasia → male hypovirilization; mouse: normal sex differentiation Males and females infertile
STAR*	8p11.2	STAR	Mitochondrial transport protein	Not applicable	Transports cholesterol to inner mitochondrial membrane	Human mutation: congenital lipoid adrenal hyperplasia; 46,XY undervirilization
SRD5A2*	2p23	5α-Reductase 2	Mitochondrial enzyme	Not applicable	Converts testosterone → DHT	5α-Reductase deficiency; 46,XY undervirilization
AR*	Xq11.2–q12	AR	Ligand-dependent nuclear receptor	AMHR, CYP19	Regulates transcription	XY mice: undervirilization of internal and external genitalia; 46,XY human mutation: androgen insensitivity syndrome
AMH*	19p13.3	AMH	Glycoprotein homodimer of TGF-β family	Mesenchymal and epithelial cells of Müllerian ducts	Ligand for AMHR; stimulates apoptosis of Müllerian duct	46,XY human mutation: Persistent Müllerian duct syndrome
AMHR2*	12q13	Type II AMH receptor (AMHR2)	Transmembrane serine/threonine kinase receptor	Mesenchymal and epithelial cells of Müllerian ducts	Receptor for AMH; stimulates apoptosis of Müllerian duct	Persistent Müllerian duct syndrome
Factors involved in ovary/female sex determination						
RSPO1*	1p34	RSPO1	Thrombospondin-like secreted activator of β-catenin	WNT4, CTNNB1	Expressed in testis, ovary, adrenals, thyroid, trachea, kidney, skin Controls expression of CTNNB1 (gene for β-catenin) in developing ovary	Mouse: XX null show partial female-to-male sex reversal, with the development of seminiferous tubules; Human: 46,XY sex reversal and palmoplantar keratosis

Continued

Table 1.1 Genetic factors with possible roles in sexual determination or differentiation—cont'd

Gene name or pseudonyms	Human gene locus	Protein name	Protein type	Genetic or cellular targets of factors	Action of factors	Effects of overexpression or underexpression of gene
WNT4*	1p36.23–p35.1	WNT4	Cysteine-rich signaling molecule/secreted growth factor	Mesonephric mesenchyme	Directs initial Müllerian duct formation in both sexes; "antitestis" factor in ovarian development	XX and XY null mice: Müllerian duct agenesis. Overexpression in XY: male-to-female sex reversal. Human 46,XY: duplication of WNT4 associated with male-to-female sex reversal
FOXL2*	3q23	FOXL2	Transcription factor	Not reported	Expressed predominantly in ovary; earliest known marker of ovarian differentiation in mammals	Goat: deletion associated with XX sex reversal. Human mutation: 46,XX gonadal dysgenesis
HOXA13*	7p15–p14	HOXA13	Homeodomain transcription factor	FGF8, BMP7	Involved in epithelial–mesenchymal interactions required for morphogenesis of terminal gut and urogenital tract, including Müllerian structures	Mouse: XX null have hypoplasia of cervix and vagina. 46,XX human mutation: hand–foot–genital syndrome with uterine malformation
Factors with possible roles in either or both sexes						
DAX1* NR0B1 AHCH	Xp21.3–p21.2	DAX1 NROB1	Orphan nuclear receptor transcription factor	RAR, RXR, STAR, CYP17A1, HSD3B2	Represses SF1 transcription; antagonizes SF1; regulates testis cord organization. Presents premature cell differentiation Dose-dependent effects	Strain-specific defects in XY mice: overexpression → testis maldevelopment and sex reversal; homozygous deletion → adrenal hypoplasia, normal testes. Human mutations: adrenal hypoplasia congenita, hypothalamic hypogonadism

Gene	Locus	Protein	Type	Expression	Function	Phenotype
WNT7A	3p25	WNT7A	Signaling molecule	Mesenchymal and epithelial cells of Müllerian ducts	XY: involved in Müllerian duct regression; XX: stimulates the development of Müllerian duct	Male mice with homozygous ceficiency of Wnt7a have retained Müllerian ducts; female Wnt7a-deficient mice have defective, though not absent, development of cviducts and uterus
DMRT1/2*	9p24.3	DMRT1 DMRT2	DM-domain transcription factors		Expressed only in genital ridge. Dose-dependent effect on postnatal testis development	XY null mice have normal prenatal testis development but abnormal postnatal testis differentiation. Human monosomy 9p: 46,XY testis maldevelopment; 46,XX primary hypogonadism

KO, knockout; NR, not reported. *Means the gene has reported mutations in humans. Many genes listed have mutations that were reported only in mice.
Reproduced with permission from Arboleda VA, Quigley CA, Vilain E. Chapter 118—Genetic basis of gonadal and genital development. In: Jameson JL, De Groot LJ, de Kretser DM, et al., eds. Endocrinology: Adult and Pediatric. 7th ed. Philadelphia: Elsevier Saunders; 2016:2051–2085.e7 [Table 118-1].

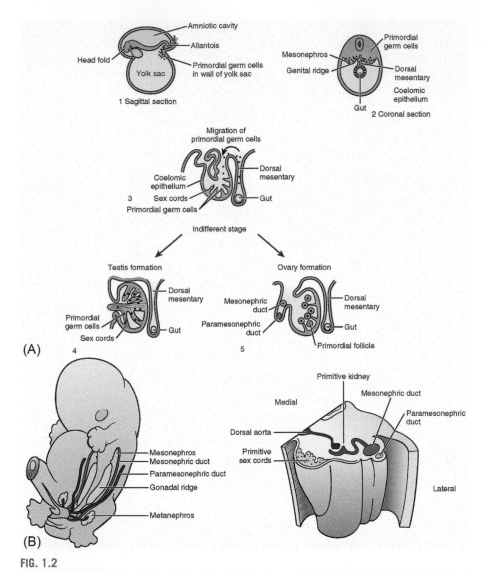

FIG. 1.2

Gonadal embryogenesis and anatomical relationships. Gonadal embryology (A) and the anatomical relationships during embryogenesis (B).

Reproduced with permission from Arboleda VA, Quigley CA, Vilain E. Chapter 118—Genetic basis of gonadal and genital development. In: Jameson JL, De Groot LJ, de Kretser DM, et al., eds. Endocrinology: Adult and Pediatric. 7th ed. Philadelphia: Elsevier Saunders; 2016:2051–2085.e7 [Figure 118-1].

Their path goes through the dorsal mesentery and the journey seems to require the influence of various genes (i.e., homeobox protein Lim-1 (*LHX1* or *Lim1*) for proper hindgut localization and WNT family member 5A (*WNT5A*) for the PGCs to receive a proper migration cue; the mutation of the latter can partly explain findings in Robinow syndrome),[12,13] the action of ligand/receptor pathways (i.e., stromal cell-derived factor

1 (Sdf1 or C–X–C motif chemokine 12 (CXCL12)/CXC receptor 4 (CXCR4) pathway),[14] an optimum collagen-I deposition in the extracellular matrix (i.e., induced by TGF-β through the activin receptor-like kinase 5 (alk5)),[15] and the help of autonomic nerve fibers migrating along with them to the same destination.[11]

The development of the genital ridge commences and proceeds in conjunction with the migration. The urogenital ridge arises as a dorsal body wall thickening that harbors populations from both the primitive mesoderm and the coelomic epithelium (viz., adrenogenital primordium).[16] The central portion—the mesonephros—of the urogenital ridge gives rise to the gonadal ridge along its ventromedial surface—which starts bulging after germ cells infiltrate it to form the primordial indifferent gonad by the end of the 5th week of intrauterine life.[17,18] Certain gene mutations can affect the development of genital ridge (i.e., and consequently risk the lack of the development of the gonads themselves in addition to some malfunctions in the adrenal and renal systems) and they include[19,20] Wilms' tumor 1 (*Wt1*), steroidogenic factor-1 (*SF1*), *Lhx1*, *Lhx9*, empty spiracles homeobox 2 (*Emx2*), and GATA-binding protein 4 (*GATA4*).

The indifferent stage, the bipotential gonad, and the gonadal differentiation

Sustainment of the morphological development of the gonads requires the presence and the influence of germ cells only in the case of the ovary (i.e., normal testicular development continues in their absence)[21]; however, both the cortex and the medulla of the indifferent gonads change according to the genotype of the fetus (i.e., cortex develop and medulla regresses in the case of the XX genotype and the medullary sex cords proliferate toward seminiferous tubules formation in the case of the XY genotype).[22] Interestingly, PGCs differentiate into male or female gametes according to the cellular environment they are placed in. For instance, female genotypic PGCs become spermatogonia when they are placed in gonads with testicular somatic cell environment (i.e., of Sertoli cell lineage) while those migrating to aberrant locations give rise to oogonia—that degenerate afterward—irrespective of their sexual genotype (i.e., though rarely they form teratomas in certain locations as the mediastinum).[1] Assumptions about the sexual identity of the gonad grow stronger as intrauterine life progresses over the weeks depending on a number of clues—which when working toward an assumption of the presence of an ovary—that include the following: lack of testicular development beyond the 7th week; the presence of oogonial meiosis around the time of the 8th week; and visualization of primordial follicles by the 16th week.[23]

Gonadal differentiation seems to rely on intricate genetic interactions between multiple upstream and downstream factors (Fig. 1.3), many of which are yet to be fully elucidated. The long-held belief that the female differentiation pathway is the default one in the absence of male factors' influences has recently started to be challenged. Consequently, for example, and in the case of female gonad determination and the hypotheses behind it, two possibilities are now entertained for the directions factor takes to achieve the determination: repression of somatic testis-inducing genes

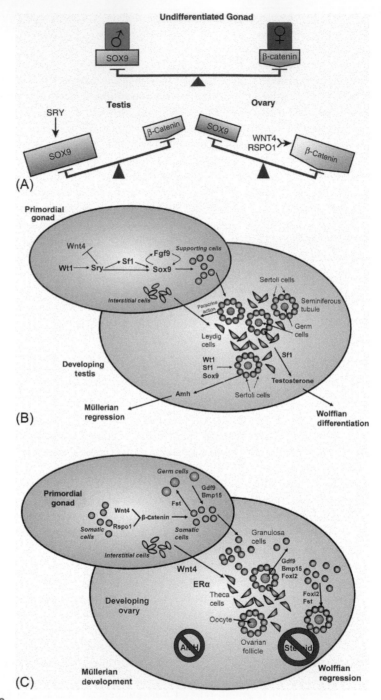

FIG. 1.3

Hypothetical models of gonadal determination. Hypothetical model of signal balance during initial sex determination in the undifferentiated gonad (A), testis determination (B), and ovary determination (C). *Arrows* denote stimulatory actions while *blunt-ended pointers* in (B) denote inhibitory actions.

Reproduced with permission from Arboleda VA, Quigley CA, Vilain E. Chapter 118—Genetic basis of gonadal and genital development. In: Jameson JL, De Groot LJ, de Kretser DM, et al., eds. Endocrinology: Adult and Pediatric. 7th ed. Philadelphia: Elsevier Saunders; 2016:2051–2085.e7 [Figure 118-3].

in addition to the activation of ovary stimulating ones as one possibility; downregulation of the same male genes while removing the repression on ovary stimulating ones as an alternate possibility.[3] It is worthy of note that no definite hypothetical model has been adopted yet even when the knowledge about possible factors keeps-on expanding.

At about the 7th week and under the influence of the autosomal gene *SRY* (sex-determining region Y)-box 9 (*SOX9*) (i.e., which gets inhibited mainly by *β-catenin* or catenin beta-1 gene (*CTNNB1*) in the case of ovary determination pathway and is upregulated by the SRY gene),[24] Sertoli cells differentiate, proliferate, and surround the arriving PGCs to form primitive sex cords while protecting the PGCs from entering meiosis prematurely (i.e., protection is vital for commitment to spermatogenesis and is mediated by degrading retinoic acid—and possibly other products—by the cytochrome p450 enzyme (Cyp26b1); mitotic arrest continues until puberty).[3,17,25] Sertoli cells promote differentiation of peritubular myoid cells and—by the 8th week—Leydig cells (i.e., both arising from primitive interstitial cells) by secreting anti-Müllerian hormone (AMH) as a paracrine factor.[3] *SRY* and other factors (i.e., transmembrane ligand ephrin-B2) influence to proper vascularization of the testes—which is characterized by early distinct arterial specification and is necessary for further transportation of testicular hormones.[26,27] From the second trimester thereafter, Sertoli cells double in number fortnightly (i.e., coupled by a parallel increase in numbers of germ and Leydig cells) resulting in a rapid increase in testicular sizes.[3] It is evident that Y-chromosome genes are necessary to maintain spermatogenesis while having extra X-chromosomes (i.e., as is the case with Klinefelter's syndrome) can result in compromised testicular development and size.[3]

An alternate developmental path is generally followed in the case of the ovary and differs from that of the testis in the following points:

- Failure of migration of PGCs results in a degenerated fibrous streak being formed (i.e., Turner syndrome).[1,21] After their successful arrival and infiltration of the secondary cortical sex cords, the medulla starts to regress and the ovaries start to become distinguishable by the 6–8th weeks. PGCs undergo vigorous mitotic duplication during that time (i.e., reaching 600,000 in number as oogonia by the 8th week); subsequently, meiosis (i.e., which is facilitated by the action of retinoic acid and possibly nonretinoic acid factors),[25] oogonial atresia, and the ongoing mitosis regulate their number until they reach a peak of at least 6 million cells by mid-gestation—at the time of formation of the first primordial follicle and breakdown of oocyte cell nests—and then decline afterward (i.e., cells entering meiosis freeze their progress at the meiosis-I phase by the 17th week to resume meiosis later in puberty).[2,8] By the 7th month, mitosis is terminated and oogonial atresia is replaced by follicular atresia which withers their number to only 700,000 primordial follicles at birth (i.e., and 300,000 by the time of puberty).[8] Fig. 1.4 provides more details about oogenesis throughout the intrauterine period.

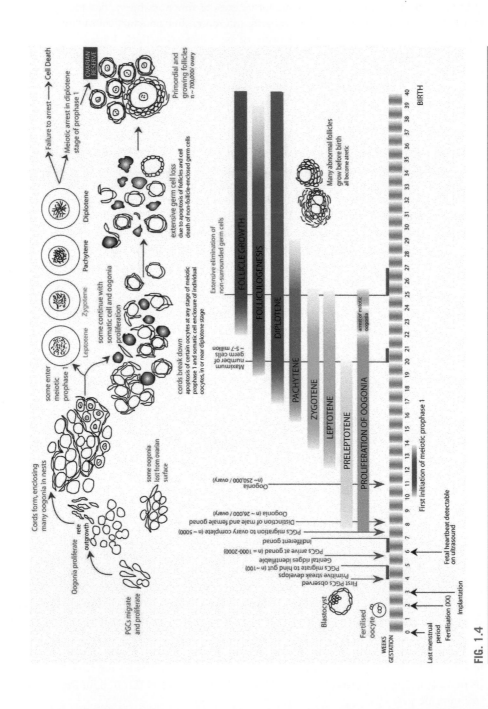

FIG. 1.4

Intrauterine fetal oogenesis timeline.

*Reproduced with permission from Hartshorne GM, Lyrakou S, Hamoda H, Oloto E, Ghafari F. Oogenesis and cell death in human prenatal ovaries:
what are the criteria for oocyte selection? Mol Hum Reprod. 2009;15(12):805–819 [Figure 1].*

- Pregranulosa cells lack *SRY* expression that allows *SOX9* to be antagonized properly and—thus—the commitment to granulosa cell lineage can occur under the influence of the *WNT4/β-catenin* pathway.[24]
- The forkhead box 2 (*Foxl2*) gene maintains such differentiation by continuous suppression of *SOX9*.[5]
- Nuclear receptor subfamily 0 group B member 1 (*NR0B1*) gene (formerly called dosage-sensitive sex reversal, adrenal hypoplasia critical region, on chromosome X, gene 1 (*DAX1*)) is a dosage-sensitive gene that needs two copies to antagonize *SOX9* and *SF1*.[28] Conversely, as suggested by its formal name, the absence of *NR0B1* gene (i.e., low dose) can potentially result in testicular dysgenesis.[29,30]
- Theca cells are the Leydig cells' female counterparts and developed from the interstitial cells under the influence of *WNT4* and *Foxl2* genes and in the absence of the effect of high levels of testosterone.[3,5,24]
- Vascularization of the ovary follows the classic angiogenic route rather than recruiting endothelial cells by breaking down mesonephric vessels.[31]

Gonadal relocation and descent (Fig. 1.5)

Testicular migration—and descent—begins around the 12th week of intrauterine life, goes through two major phases (viz., transabdominal and inguinoscrotal phases), and ends with the successful intra-scrotal positioning by the 32nd gestational week.[18,32] In addition to the increase in the intraabdominal pressure and the passive change in position that occurs as a result of elongation of the trunk and enlargement of the pelvis (i.e., both phenomena are common to both sexes), the descent is aided in males by the secretory products of Leydig cells (including testosterone and insulin-like factor 3 (Insl3) and anti-Müllerian hormone (AMH)) that result—first—in the simultaneous regression of the craniosuspensory ligament and differentiation of the gubernaculum (i.e., to develop muscular tissue) and then the contraction of the latter to guide the testes through the inguinal canal (i.e., that contracts around the spermatic cord afterward preventing inguinal hernia)[33] and into the scrotum—a process that the genitofemoral nerve is hypothesized to mediate through the action of calcitonin gene-related peptide (CGRP).[18,32,34] Mutations in the *INSL3* gene or its receptor gene (viz., relaxin/insulin-like family peptide receptor 2 [*RXFP2*], aka leucine-rich repeat-containing G protein-coupled receptor 8 [*LGR8*] or G protein-coupled receptor affecting testis descent [*GREAT*]), deficient Insl3 production, or fetal androgen insufficiency/resistance are associated with cryptorchidism in humans.[35]

In females, the craniosuspensory ligament remains intact (i.e., which later gives rise to the ovarian suspensory ligament) while the gubernaculum remains undifferentiated (i.e., which later gives rise to the round ligament of the ovary [superior part] and that of the uterus [inferior part] which is anchored to both labia majora).[1] Therefore, the ovaries only undergo a caudal shift to become positioned lateral to the kidneys.[34]

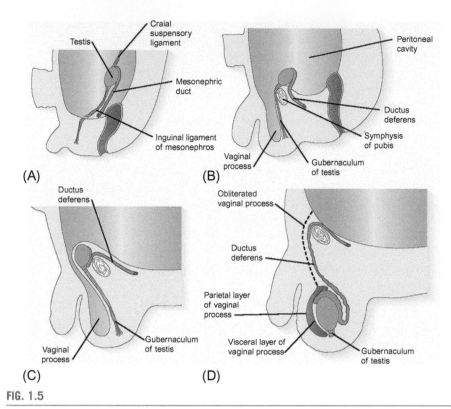

FIG. 1.5

Fetal testicular descent. Figure outlines testicular descent steps during the intrauterine life. (A) During the 2nd gestational month. (B) During the 3rd month. (C) During the 7th month. (D) At term.

Reproduced with permission from Carlson BM. Chapter 16: Urogenital system. Part II: development of the body systems. In: Carlson BM, ed. Human Embryology and Developmental Biology. 5th ed. Philadelphia: Elsevier Saunders; 2014:376–407 [Fig. 16.35].

Sexual duct differentiation (Fig. 1.6)

At week 4 of gestation, the indifferent stage of sexual duct differentiation begins as the mesonephric duct (aka Wolffian duct) forms from the lateral nephrotomes (i.e., intermediate mesoderm segments), followed 2 weeks later by the emergence of the paramesonephric duct (aka Müllerian duct) as an invagination of the urogenital ridge's surface epithelium.[3,17] After another 2 weeks, the testosterone secreted by the Leydig cells induces the differentiation of the Wolffian ducts into the epididymides (cranial segment), vasa deferentia, and seminal vesicles (lower segment) over the succeeding 4 weeks (i.e., dihydrotestosterone (DHT) does not influence the process as evident from the lack of 5α-reductase 2 enzyme expression in Wolffian ducts during differentiation).[3,36] A simultaneous process of defeminization takes place where the Müllerian ducts regress under the effect of the AMH to completely disappear by the 11th week

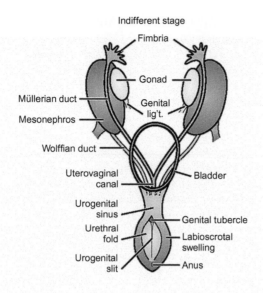
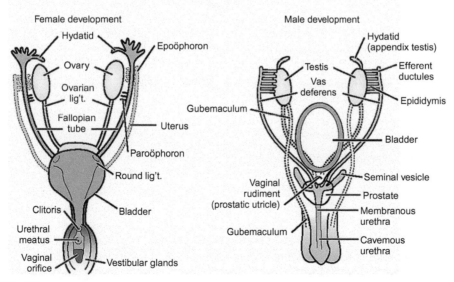

FIG. 1.6

Embryologic sexual duct differentiation. Indifferent internal genitalia (*top*). Female differentiation (*bottom left*). Male differentiation (*bottom right*). *Dotted lines* represent obliterated structures.

(i.e., AMH—or Müllerian inhibitory substance (MIS)—produced by Sertoli cells and the mechanism is mainly an apoptotic one).[36] Both hormones might be primarily acting in a paracrine manner since unilateral testicular absence leads to ipsilateral persistence of the Müllerian structures and residual development of Wolffian ones[36,37]; inactivating mutations of *AMH* gene or *AMH type II* receptor defects can also negatively impact the functions of AMH (i.e., persistent Müllerian duct syndrome (PMDS) while overexpression in females leads to blind vagina and the absence of oviducts.[10,36,38] Conversely in normal 46,XX females, the absence of the AMH allows the Müllerian ducts to continue their differentiation into fallopian tubes (cranial portions), uterus, cervix, and the upper third of the vagina (i.e., the lower portion originates from the urogenital sinus) while the absence of the testosterone prevents the differentiation of the Wolffian ducts (i.e., thus only nonfunctioning remnants can persist).[36]

Some genetic defects can potentially result in the complete absence of reproductive tracts including the null mutation of *Emx2*, *Lim-1*, and paired box 2 (*Pax2*) genes; *WNT4* and *WNT7A* mutations are accompanied with the masculinization of reproductive tracts in females in the case of the former and with Müllerian regression failure in males (causing obstructive sterility)—and Müllerian defective differentiation in females—in the case of the latter.[10,39] Homeobox-containing genes (*HOX*) are very important in the specification of various male and female tract parts and are expressed from top downward with increasing numbering (i.e., *Hoxd10–13* or its *Hoxa* paralogues) such that mutations of—for example—*Hoxa10* leads to the transformation of the cranial uterine part into a fallopian tube in females and ductus deferens to epididymis in males.[1,40] In humans, *HOXA13* mutation leads to the hand–foot–genital syndrome (aka Guttmacher syndrome) where there are Müllerian defects in females and hypospadias in males (i.e., in addition to limb abnormalities).[41]

External genitalia and other accessory glands differentiation

The external genitalia of both sexes develop indifferently until the 8th week of gestation (i.e., the start of testosterone secretion); before then, an initial elevation called the genital tubercle is formed—at the cloacal membrane's cranial end and possibly guided by fibroblast growth factor 8 (*Fgf8*) gene—by the 4th week (i.e., primordial penis or clitoris), and then the urethral (medial) and labioscrotal (lateral) folds (i.e., primordial labia minora/penile foreskin and labia majora/scrotum, respectively) flank the urogenital groove by the 6th week and the indifferent stage appears largely hormonal-independent.[3,18]

The presence of DHT (i.e., converted by the action of 5α-reductase enzyme on testosterone) and its action on androgen receptor (AR) in the target tissues (i.e., external genitalia and some accessory glands like the prostate) is the deciding factor for masculinization of them (i.e., in the case of deficiency of DHT—or in the case of resistance like in androgen insensitivity syndrome—the external genitalia develop down the female pathway).[3] By the 12th week of gestation, those going down the path of masculinization complete the process of male sexual differentiation of the external genitalia (i.e., genital tubercle elongation as penis, urethral folds ventral fusion as penile urethra, and labioscrotal folds midline fusion as scrotum) and the prostate (i.e., develops from the urogenital sinus after the vesicovaginal septum formation is inhibited)—penile enlargement, however, continues further in the third trimester (i.e., which seems quite incomplete in cases of fetal hypopituitarism—or luteinizing hormone receptor β (LHβ) mutations—since the androgen production is less dependent on the maternal chorionic gonadotropin (CG) stimulation in the third trimester)[42,43] and the whole penile enlargement appears to be under the regulation of *HOX*, *FGF*, and Sonic hedgehog (*Shh*) genes. In the absence of proper androgen stimulation (i.e., female, androgen deficiency, or androgen resistance), the external genitalia continue down the female pathway and also complete the differentiation by the 12th week as follows: genital tubercle slightly enlarges as clitoris, urogenital sinus remains open, vesicovaginal septum forms, urethral folds become labia minora, and labioscrotal folds become labia majora (i.e., minor labial fusions lead to the formation of mons pubis (anteriorly) and posterior commissure (posteriorly)).[3] Urethral and urogenital sinus outgrowths produce urethral/para-urethral glands and great vestibular glands, respectively.[18] Table 1.2 illustrates homologous parts of the urogenital system of both genders.

Table 1.2 homologous parts of the urogenital system of both genders.

Indifferent structure	Male derivative	Female derivative
Genital ridge	Testis	Ovary
Primordial germ cells	Spermatozoa	Ova
Sex cords	Seminiferous tubules (Sertoli cells)	Follicular (granulosa) cells
Mesonephric tubules	Efferent ductules	Oöphoron
	Paradidymis	Paroöphoron
Mesonephric (Wolffian) ducts	Appendix of epididymis	Appendix of ovary
	Epididymal duct	Gartner's duct
	Ductus deferens	
	Ejaculatory duct	
	Seminal vesicles	
Mesonephric ligaments	Gubernaculum testis	Round ligament of ovary
		Round ligament of uterus
Paramesonephric (Müllerian) ducts	Appendix of testis	Uterine tubes
	Prostate utricle	Uterus
		Upper vagina
Definitive urogenital sinus (lower part)	Penile urethra	Lower vagina
	Bulbourethral glands	Vaginal vestibule
Early urogenital sinus (upper part)	Urinary bladder	Urinary bladder
	Prostatic urethra	Urethra
	Prostate gland	Glands of Skene
Genital tubercle	Penis	Clitoris
Genital folds	Floor of penile urethra	Labia minora
Genital swellings	Scrotum	Labia majora

Anatomy of the male reproductive system

The male reproductive system is anatomically divided into internal and external genitalia. The internal genitalia include the gonads (testes), the spermatic cords, and the accessory organs and glands while the external genitalia constitute a penis and a scrotum.

 The role of the male genital system ensures the production of enough viable male gametes, their successful transportation, and the regulated secretion of male sex hormones in a manner that leads to acceptable sexual desire and potency.

Testes and spermatogenesis

The male gonads (testes) are the most important component of the male reproductive system since it is the sole source of the gametes and the main source of male sex hormone (testosterone).[44] As per the currently available literature, each testis is an oval-shaped firm organ with measurements ranging from 3.7 to 5.1 cm in terms of length, 2 to 3.1 cm in terms of width, and 3 to 5.2 cm in the anteroposterior diameter; measurements determined clinically are useful for estimating volume (i.e., by incorporating them in equations) and can be used as cutoffs to help diagnose certain syndromes (i.e., < 3.5 cm longest diameter Klinefelter's syndrome[45]).[46–49] Additionally, each normally possesses a weight that ranges from 12 to 26 g and a volume that ranges from 14.8 to 28 mL[44,49] (i.e., clinically[48,50] or a US measured range of 10–17 mL[47,51]).

 For spermatogenesis to proceed properly, the temperature of the testes has to be held at a level 3–4°C lower than the cores and this is normally facilitated by several factors: their position in the scrotum outside the body (i.e., which is continuously corrected by the cremasteric muscle according to testicular and scrotal temperatures), the special characteristics of the scrotal skin (see later), and the pampiniform venous plexus maintained countercurrent exchange mechanism (i.e., by surrounding the testicular artery with their colder blood). Conditions that increase such temperature result in impaired spermatogenesis (i.e., cryptorchidism and frequent hot baths; the latter can cause a temporary effect with a recovery of at least 3 months).[33,49,52]

 The testes usually lie obliquely suspended by the spermatic cords in the scrotum and buried inside three layers of coverings (i.e., ordered from outside inward): a peritoneum-like tunica vaginalis (i.e., covering all but the testicular posterior aspect; it's the extension of the processus vaginalis whose incomplete closure predisposes to indirect inguinal hernia and hydroceles), the fibrous tunica albuginea, (i.e., which creates the mediastinum testis) and the vascular tunica vasculosa (i.e., which is in-line with all surfaces of the testis and tunica albuginea's septations going into it).[33,49] Fig. 1.7 provides an illustration of the testes and their surrounding relationships.

Microstructure

Each testis is subdivided, roughly, into 250 lobules by the septa extending from the mediastinum testis and each has up to 4 convoluted seminiferous tubules (i.e., they contribute to approximately 80% of testicular volume and have a diameter of

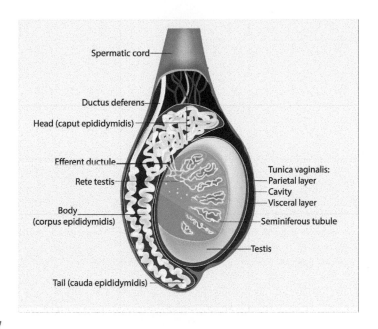

FIG. 1.7

Cross-sectional illustration of the testis and its surrounding structures.

Original image at Shutterstock, by Sakurra, and available at https://www.shutterstock.com/image-vector/
testicles-testes-illustration-cross-section-testis-676139677.

around 200 μm with a total length of 0.25–0.6 km) with interspersing interstitial tissue (i.e., containing the testosterone-secreting Leydig cells, mast cells, and macrophage together with nerve fibers and vascular structures). Seminiferous tubules are lined internally by Sertoli cells (i.e., responsible for maintaining a blood-testis barrier, phagocytosis, and other—mostly secretory—functions; their number does not affect the spermatogenic cycle length itself but is essential for its normal capacity[53]) and has spermatozoa going through the different stages of their development. Spermatogenic cells are more concentrated at the highly convoluted portions and are completely replaced in the lack of such coiling by cuboidal epithelium—at short tubuli recti—followed by flat epithelium (i.e., at the anastomosis of tubuli recti to form rete testis where sperms are concentrated after the intratubular fluid is absorbed). From the rete testis, at least seven ciliated efferent ductules relay the spermatozoa to the caput of the epididymis.[44,49]

Spermatogenesis (Fig. 1.8)

In human males, spermatogenesis is a strictly organized process that yields around 1 spermatozoon per heartbeat daily[54] (i.e., or 4.25 million spermatozoa per gram per day on average). The process entails three phases: an initial mitotic—or proliferative—phase where spermatogonia either replenish the stem cell pool or continue the differentiation toward mature spermatozoa production (i.e., and hence, they are termed

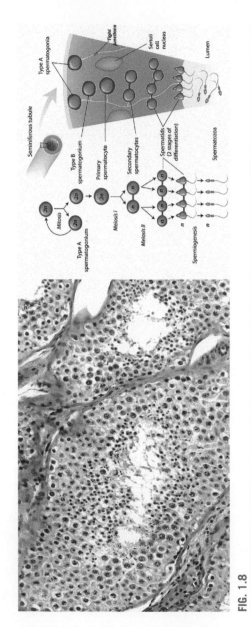

FIG. 1.8

Spermatogenesis and cross section of the testis and seminiferous tubules.

Original images at Shutterstock: Right is by Alila Medical Media and is available at https://www.shutterstock.com/image-illustration/spermatogenesis-process-sperm-production-male-seminiferous-116875789; left is by David A. Litman and is available at https://www.shutterstock.com/image-photo/cross-section-human-testis-showing-seminiferous-1091292833.

type A and B), a meiotic phase where haploid spermatids are the product, and finally spermiogenesis where the maturation of spermatids into spermatozoa takes place (i.e., followed by spermiation during which spermatozoa get released into seminiferous tubules' lumens).[33,53] Given that the whole process (i.e., from mitosis to spermatozoal release) takes 60–70 days to finish[55] (i.e., not counting the epididymal transit time), it is reasonably expected that the effects of external insults—or contraceptives—are to become noticeable months after the damage (i.e., as a low sperm count).

Vascular supply, neural supply, and lymphatic drainage

Three main arteries carry the role of supplying the testes with blood: testicular artery (i.e., internal spermatic artery which has the most contribution: two-thirds), cremasteric arteries, and vasal artery.[56,57] This collateral vascular supply ensures testicular survival during surgical correction of high undescended testis (i.e., main testicular artery ligation done during orchiopexy).[33] Vascular drainage of the testis starts off as testicular veins from its posterior aspect and from very complex anastomoses with each other to form the pampiniform venous plexus that ascends into the spermatic cord anterior to the vas deferens to pour into three to four veins inside the inguinal canal and that then merges into one testicular vein (aka internal spermatic vein and they have one-way valves that can cause varicoceles if they have any defects or if compressed externally[58]) to drain either into the inferior vena cava (in case of the right vein where it joins at an acute angle) or into the left renal vein (in case of the left vein where it joins at a right angle).[49] The right testis drains mainly into the interaortocaval and paracaval lymph nodes (i.e., sometimes it drains into the left para-aortic ones) while the left drains into the left para-aortic and interaortocaval nodes; this route is common for testicular metastasis.[33] Nerve supply accompanies testicular vessels and vas deferens and originates from renal, aortic, and pelvic plexuses, and some fibers can cross over to the contralateral plexus (i.e., possibly explaining the affection of the healthy testis in the event of the other having a pathology).[59]

The epididymis

The epididymis starts posterolaterally to the testis, separated from it only laterally by the sinus epididymis (i.e., cases of nonfusion have been described in those with cryptorchidism[60]), as the caput of the epididymis from which stems a corpus and then a cauda that connect to the convoluted part of vas deferens.[49] Its duct is 3–4 m in length, surrounded by smooth muscles that produce rhythmic contractions (i.e., supplied by sympathetic inferior spermatic nerve fibers[61]) and is covered by the tunica vaginalis.[62] The lining-ciliated epithelium absorbs testicular fluid and helps sperm transfer and maturation (i.e., a journey of an average 12-day duration[63]).

The vas deferens

The vas deferens relays the sperms to the urethra and its cells appear to be able to exert other functions beneficial to them (i.e., absorptive or secretory functions carried out by a complex epithelium[64]). It starts as a tortuous structure of 2–3 cm in length, ascends inside the spermatic cord into the inguinal canal, and then leaves the testicular vessels—just lateral to the inferior epigastric vessels—at the internal ring. Finally, it moves medial to the pelvic wall structures to become the ampulla of the vas at the base of the prostate to unite with the seminal vesicle's duct and end as the ejaculatory duct[49] (i.e., which when rarely obstructed causes oligospermia). The tube is 30–35 cm in length, has a diameter of 2–3 mm, and interestingly has a thick three-layered muscular wall giving it the highest muscle to lumen ratio in comparison with any other hollow tube in the body (i.e., 10:1). The main arterial supply is the vassal artery, main destination of venous drainage is the pelvic plexus, and main lymphatic drainage destination is the external and internal iliac nodes. Its muscles are mainly supplied by postganglionic sympathetic nerve fibers.[61]

The accessory glands

Three accessory glands help enrich the seminal fluid with nutrients and important factors, in descending order of contribution; they are the seminal vesicles (i.e., 13 mL average in volume, at least 50% of the ejaculate volume is supplied by it and is rich in fructose), the prostate (i.e., around 20% of ejaculate volume which is rich in sugars and zinc), bulbourethral and periurethral glands (viz., Cowper's and Littre's glands secreting mainly mucus for lubrication).[49,61,65] Both the seminal vesicles and the prostate receive dual autonomic nerve supply from the pelvis plexus.

The penis (Fig. 1.9)

The penis has a perineum-attached radix and a free pendulous skin-covered shaft[49] and is anchored to the symphysis pubis by two suspensory ligaments, and its adult form has the following ranges of measurements on average[47,48,50]: a stretched penile length (SPL) of 8.5–11.9 cm and a width of 2.7–3.5 cm. Internally, the shaft consists of three spongy erectile bodies (viz., two corpora cavernosa dorsally and one corpus spongiosum ventrally), the penile urethra, and the accompanying neurovascular structures, and fascia (i.e., tunica albuginea covers the corpora under the cover of Buck's and Colles' fascia).[49] At the radix, the two corpora cavernosa are anchored to the ischiopubic rami—as the tapered crura penis—while the corpus spongiosum forms the bulbospongiosus muscle proximally between them and enlarges distally to form the glans of the penis (i.e., separated from the shaft by the corona—the only gland-harboring skin that produces smegma[61]—and is covered by the loose retractable prepuce).

Vascular supply, neural supply, and lymphatic drainage

The internal pudendal artery is the main artery that supplies the ischiocavernosus and bulbospongiosus through the perianal artery and the rest of the penis through the common penile artery and its three branches.[49] Three systems of veins are draining the penis and end either into the great saphenous vein (i.e., in case of superficial system), into prostatic plexus (i.e., in case of intermediate system), or into internal pudendal vein (i.e., in case of deep system). Lymph is drained into superficial inguinal,

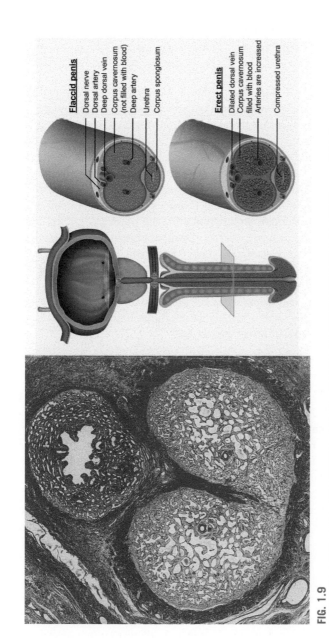

FIG. 1.9

Penile internal structure (flaccid and erect) with cross section.

Original images at Shutterstock: Right is by medical stocks and is available at https://www.shutterstock.com/image-vector/penis-anatomy-cross-section-medical-3d-1308540718; left is by MriMan and is available at https://www.shutterstock.com/image-photo/cross-section-penis-tissue-microscopic-view-286437428.

Flaccid penis

Dorsal nerve
Dorsal artery
Deep dorsal vein
Corpus cavernosum (not filled with blood)
Deep artery
Urethra
Corpus spongiosum

Erect penis

Dilated dorsal vein
Corpus cavernosum filled with blood
Arteries are increased
Compressed urethra

deep inguinal, external, and internal iliac nodes. Cavernous nerve is the main autonomic neural supply (i.e., causes erectile dysfunction when damaged as in radical prostatectomy operations) while the dorsal nerve of the penis (i.e., arising from the pelvis plexus) and some perineal nerve small branches are the main sensory supplies (i.e., giving the glans a rich free nerve ending innervation).[49,61]

The scrotum

The scrotum is the multiple-layered, bi-compartmental sac that surrounds the testes (i.e., that are fixed to its wall by the gubernaculum) and the spermatic cords.[49] The layers include: the internal spermatic fascia (i.e., loosely attached to the tunica vaginalis), cremasteric and external spermatic fascia, dartos muscle, and the skin. The scrotal skin is thin and varies from smooth to rugated (i.e., as per the dartos muscle's contraction degree), fat-free, hair containing, and rich in glands (i.e., sebaceous and sweat) and sensory innervation (i.e., that responds to stimulation and temperature and is supplied by ilioinguinal nerve, genital branch of genitofemoral nerve, scrotal branches of the perineal nerve, and the perineal branch of the posterior femoral cutaneous nerve). The scrotal arterial supply is fulfilled by the external pudendal branches of the femoral artery, scrotal branches of the internal pudendal artery, and a cremasteric branch from the inferior epigastric artery. Temperature regulation is facilitated by the vessel arrangement and the presence of arteriovenous anastomoses. Lymphatic drainage ends in the ipsilateral superficial inguinal nodes of each compartment with no crossing of the median raphe.

Anatomy of the female reproductive system

The female reproductive system is anatomically divided into internal and external genitalia. The internal genitalia comprise the upper genital tract (i.e., uterus, cervix, fallopian tubes, and upper vagina) and the ovaries while the external genitalia (aka the vulva) comprise the mons pubis, labia majora and labia minora, the clitoris, the vaginal vestibule, and its associated bulb and glands.[66]

The role of the female genital system includes the regular production of oocytes for spermatozoa to fertilize at timely intervals in addition to the preparation of a suitable environment for the migration of sperms and successful fetal growth and delivery. Such roles extend to include the regulated secretion of female sex hormones that are vital to orchestrating menstruation, parturition, delivery, and libido.

The ovaries

The ovaries are two dull-white oval-shaped bodies, suspended near the lateral pelvic wall by the mesovarium (i.e., that connects to the posterior aspect of the broad ligament of the uterus), the infundibulopelvic ligament, and the ovarian ligament[67]; each is 2.5–5 cm long, 1.5–3 cm wide, and 0.6–1.5 cm thick in a nonpregnant state (i.e., dimensions are those of mature women and they double during pregnancy and diminish greatly after menopause).[67,68] Their normal surface has scarrings representative of successive corpora luteal degenerations (i.e., surfaces are smooth before first ovulation).[67]

In adult nonpregnant females, the ovaries lie in the ovarian fossa and relate to various structures as follows: posteriorly to retroperitoneal structures (i.e., ureter, obturator structures, uterine artery, and the internal iliac vessels); anteriorly to broad ligament, medially to the uterus, uterine vessels, and the rectum; laterally to the parietal peritoneum and pelvic wall; superiorly to end of the fallopian tubal ends, the fimbria, ileocecal junction with the appendix on the right side and the sigmoid colon on the left; and inferiorly to the ovarian ligament (inferomedially) and the pelvic floor.[67] The knowledge of surface anatomy helps to provide proper shielding for the ovaries during radiological procedures (i.e., just below the iliac crest/umbilicus, above the symphysis pubis, and medial to the anterior superior iliac spine).[69] The position shifts upward during pregnancy where ovaries become completely abdominal structures superolateral to the gravid uterus.[67] Additionally, accessory ovaries can be found along the course of their descent, in labia majora, in the gubernacula, or in the mesovarium.[67]

Microstructure (Fig. 1.10)

The ovarian surface is covered by a single-layered, dull-white, cuboidal epithelium (aka germinal epithelium which is a misnomer) which is coated with the shiny smooth continuous mesovarium (i.e., separated from it by a white line) and overlays the tunica albuginea.[23,67] Below that layer, the ovary divides into two regions: a cortex that occupies the most portion of the postpubertal ovary and a medulla.[67] Various structures are embedded in the cortical stroma (i.e., which consists of collagen fibers and fusiform fibroblast-like cells) including follicles (i.e., oocyte-containing complexes) at various stages of development (viz., primordial, primary, secondary, and tertiary—or Graafian—follicles), corpora lutea, and other degenerative bodies.[67] The medulla is highly vascular and is arranged distinctively into a central stromal part and the hilum which is the point of attachment of the ovary to the mesovarium and has nervous structures, blood vessels, and Leydig cell-like cells (viz., hilus cells) that are LH- or hCG-responsive and are able to secrete androgens (i.e., testosterone).[67,70]

Vascular supply, neural supply, and lymphatic drainage

Each ovary is mainly supplied by the ovarian artery—through the mesovarium—that originates from the abdominal aorta just beneath the origin of renal arteries; the ovarian artery gives two terminal branches and one of them goes to the ovary (i.e., the other enters the broad ligament of the uterus to supply the ipsilateral fallopian tube).[67] The pampiniform venous plexus emerging from each ovary gives off two veins that accompany the ovarian artery upward where the left pair enters the left renal vein and the right pair enters the superior vena cava; lymphatic drainage follows those veins to pour into the para-aortic lymph nodes (i.e., drainage pours into the inguinal nodes on rare occasions).[67]

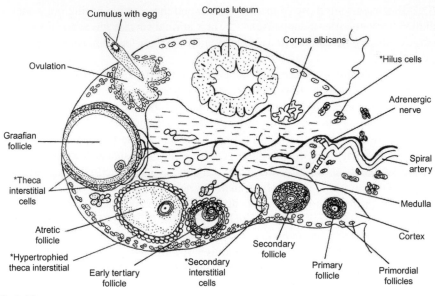

FIG. 1.10

Microstructure of the ovary during the reproductive period.

Reproduced with permission from Erickson GF, Magoffin DA, Dyer CA, Hofeditz C. The ovarian androgen producing cells: a review of structure/function relationships. Endocr Rev. 1985;6(3): 371–399 [Fig. 1].

The ovaries are supplied neurologically by ovarian plexuses that receive their autonomic innervation as follows: upper portion receives supply from renal and aortic plexuses and lower portion receives supply from both superior and inferior hypogastric plexuses.[67] These plexuses provide postganglionic sympathetic fibers (supplied by T-10 and T-11 spinal nerves) and preganglionic parasympathetic fibers while receiving visceral afferent fibers.[71]

Upper genital tract (uterus, cervix, and fallopian tubes)

The uterus is a thick-walled, hollow, muscular structure that opens into the vagina, receives both fallopian tubes (aka uterine tubes), and is positioned between the rectum (posterior to it) and the urinary bladder (anterior to it) (i.e., it is mobile with a position that changes according to the distension of the bladder or the rectum).[67] It divides into a corpus uteri (i.e., the muscular upper two-thirds) and the cervix uteri (i.e., the fibrous lower third) and is usually anteverted in relation to the vagina (i.e., except in 10%–15%) while its body is usually anteflexed in relation to its cervix (Fig. 1.11).[67]

The adult nonpregnant corpus uteri have a cavity of 6 cm in the largest diameter, receives the uterine tubes at the uterine cornua (i.e., to which relates both round and ovarian ligaments inferiorly), and is covered by the peritoneum that reflects in folds on its surfaces as follows: anteriorly it reflects on to the bladder wall at the internal os level at the uterovesical fold (i.e., creating the vesicouterine pouch), posteriorly it

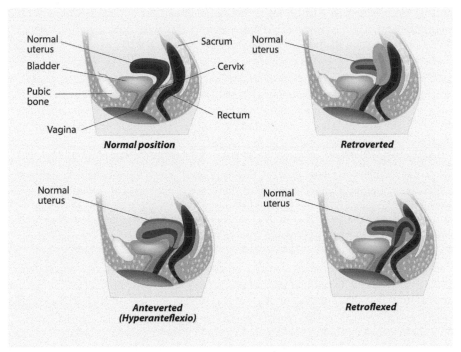

Normal uterus — Sacrum

Bladder — Cervix

Pubic bone

Vagina — Rectum

Normal position

Normal uterus

Retroverted

Normal uterus

Anteverted (Hyperanteflexio)

Normal uterus

Retroflexed

FIG. 1.11

Different positions of the uterus.

*Original images at Shutterstock, by Designua and is available at https://www.shutterstock.com/
image-illustration/uterine-position-normal-uterus-rests-on-170114252.*

reflects on to the rectal wall at the level of the cervicovaginal junction (i.e., creating the rectouterine pouch), and laterally, it forms the broad ligament that extends to the pelvic wall (i.e., and through which extends the 10–12-cm-long muscular round ligament that connects the uterine cornu to the labium majus); its wall is triple-layered and has a mucosa, myometrium (smooth muscles), and an adventitia.[67]

The cervix in nonpregnant adults is a cylindrical, fibroelastic (i.e., with less than 10% smooth muscles in its wall), 2.5-cm-long structure that connects to the body through the isthmus (i.e., its narrow upper third that becomes the lower uterine segment in pregnancy after being taken up) and projects into the vagina where it opens as a circular aperture (i.e., or the external os; which becomes a transverse slit after birth); the cervix is related to the bladder anteriorly (i.e., separated from it by the parametrium), posteriorly to the rectum, and is attached to pelvic bones by the uterosacral (posteriorly), transverse cervical (laterally), and the pubocervical ligaments (anteriorly).[66,67]

The fallopian tubes attach to the uterine body at each superior angle of the uterine cavity (i.e., uterine os); each tube continues laterally upward to end at the abdominal os, is approximately 10 cm long, and can be divided into four parts: the intramural part (0.7 mm wide and 1 cm in long), the rounded isthmus (1–5 mm wide and 3 cm long), the ampulla (i.e., widest part where fertilization takes place and is 1 cm wide and 5 cm long), and the infundibulum with its fimbriae (i.e., finger-like 1-mm-wide folds with the ovarian fimbria being the longest of them).[66,67] The tubal walls generally have three layers: inner columnar ciliated epithelium (necessary for transporting the fertilized egg to the uterine cavity, which can take around 3 days to successfully be carried out), a middle muscular layer, and a surrounding serious peritoneal coat.[66,72] The mesosalpinx is attached to each tube's inferior surface and the fimbriae protrude from its lateral end.[67]

Various congenital anomalies arise from the failure of fusion of the Müllerian ducts (i.e., which has many degrees resulting in different anomalies) the lightest of which is a nonpear-shaped uterus and the most of extreme of which is a septate vagina, duplication of cervix, duplicated uterus with single fallopian tube each.[1,73]

Vascular supply, neural supply, and lymphatic drainage

The main arterial supply to the uterus is the uterine artery (i.e., originating from the internal iliac artery) which gives off a branch that runs tortuously over the uterine body upward in the broad ligament anastomozing with the ovarian artery in the end and another that descends supplying the cervix and anastomozing with the vaginal artery; branches from uterine artery also become tortuous within the uterine wall (i.e., helicine arteries) and can straighten in pregnancy when the uterus expands.[67] Uterine veins drain the uterus into the internal iliac veins and lymph drains into the external iliac, the internal iliac, and the obturator lymph nodes (i.e., though the fundus may occasionally drain into the para-aortic nodes as is the case with the ovaries).[67]

The fallopian tubes receive arterial supply from both uterine and ovarian arteries: their medial two-thirds are supplied by uterine arteries while their lateral thirds are supplied by the ovarian arteries; venous and lymphatic drainage follows the arterial supplies (i.e., similar to that of the ovary for the lateral third and that of the uterus for the medial two-thirds).[67]

Both the uterus and the tubes are supplied by the inferior hypogastric plexus that gives off sympathetic fibers (T12–L1) and parasympathetic fibers (S2–S4) that relay in the paracervical ganglia; they are important for regulating uterine contractions and vasoconstriction or dilation.[71,74] The uterine tubes are innervated in their lateral halves by fibers from the vagus nerve and the superior hypogastric plexuses (T10–L2).[67,75]

The vagina

The vagina is a 6–12-cm-long fibromuscular tube extending from the vestibular opening to the uterus (i.e., where it surrounds the cervix in continuous recesses called fornices); the vaginal opening in the vestibular area can expand to accommodate large sizes during labor and intercourse.[67] Vaginal walls are collapsed on each other (i.e., giving a transverse slit appearance)—giving an "H" shape on transverse section (i.e., and an "S" shape on longitudinal section)—and have various important relationships[67,76]: the anterior wall (i.e., about 7.5 cm long) supports the bladder base with its upper portion and the urethra distally (i.e., which is embedded in it) with its lower portion; the posterior wall (i.e., about 9 cm long) supports the rectum superiorly—which is separated from it by the recto-uterine pouch and Denonvilliers' fascia—and contacts the fibromuscular perineal body inferiorly (i.e., separating it from the anal canal). Vaginal segments get support from muscles and ligaments differently[67]: upper vagina is supported by the levator ani muscle (i.e., claimed to be the true "constrictor cunni"),[66] transverse cervical ligament, and uterosacral ligament; mid-vagina is supported by a U-shaped pubovaginalis muscle; lower vagina is supported by the bulbospongiosus. The hymen is a thin mucous membrane of various shapes (i.e., with openings of annular, semilunar, cribriform, or completely imperforate which is detected as hematocolpos after puberty) that guards the vaginal entrance and does not serve any real function (i.e., except as an embryonic remnant)[66]; an absent hymen, however, has been linked to vaginal agenesis that appears to be associated with Mayer–Rokitansky–Kuster–Hauser (MRKH) syndrome (i.e., together with unilateral renal agenesis and other Müllerian duct anomalies), Klippel–Feil syndrome, and other congenital anomalies.[77] The vagina is lined by a nonkeratinized stratified squamous epithelium and its wall has two other layers[78]: a middle tunica muscularis with an external longitudinal and inner circular smooth muscle layers and a covering adventitious layer formed of collagen and elastin.

Vascular supply, neural supply, and lymphatic drainage

The vagina receives its vascular supply mainly from the internal iliac artery in the form of its two azygos vaginal arterial branches (i.e., though other nearby branches may occasionally contribute) and drains by the vaginal plexuses through the vaginal veins and into the internal iliac veins.[67] Lymphatic drainage follows three routes[67]: upper vessels pour into the internal and external iliac nodes, middle vessels pour into the internal iliac nodes, and lower vessels pour into the superficial inguinal lymph nodes.

The upper and lower vagina receive their neural supply differently where the pelvic splanchnic nerves (mainly S2 and S3) supply the former and the pudendal nerve (S2–S4) supplies the latter.[67] The G-spot is a nerve-rich area in close proximity to the clitoris, is important for orgasm, and facilitates vaginal blood engorgement through entrapment[79]; its nature and existence have long been controversial even though lots of scientific evidence that supports its presence is accumulating continuously.[79,80]

The vulva (Fig. 1.12)

The mons pubis is the coarse hair-bearing prominent area of skin and fatty tissue overlaying the symphysis pubis and other pubic bones that is bounded superiorly by the pubic hairline and inferiorly by the clitoris.[67] The labia majora are two longitudinal skin folds that span the area between the mons pubis and the perineum, fuse together as the anterior commissure anteriorly while merging into nearby skin without fusion posteriorly (i.e., at the posterior commissure), and contain smooth

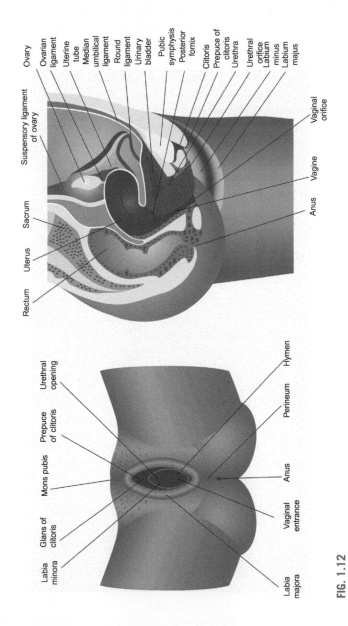

FIG. 1.12

Illustration of the female external genitalia (front and cross section with relationships).

Original images at Shutterstock, by Lotan and is available at https://www.shutterstock.com/image-vector/ female-urogenital-system-anatomy-reproductive-median-499931977.

muscles (i.e., dartos muscle-like), fatty tissue, vessels, nerves, and glands (i.e., and the insertion of the round ligament); their inner surface has sebaceous glands while the outer one is hairy and pigmented.[67]

Situated between both labia majora are another two smaller fat-free folds—each measuring 3–4 cm in length—called labia minora.[66] Each fold extends posteriorly to the fourchette and anterior to surround the clitoris by fusing to form the prepuce above its glans or its frenulum below it.[66] The medial surface is rich in sebaceous glands and both folds contain numerous nerve endings, vascular erectile structures, and connective tissue.[66,67]

The clitoris is the homologous structure to the male erectile penile ones. It has three parts: a root, a body (i.e., palpable through the skin), and a glans (i.e., the fifth of which is usually visible) and consists internally of two corpora cavernosa (Fig. 1.13).[76] The corpora diverge with the pubic rami forming the crura under the cover of the ischiocavernosus muscle proximally[76]; the glans covers the corpora's distal part, is 3.7–6.5 mm in longitudinal diameter (i.e., length), 2.4–4.4 mm in transverse diameter (i.e., width), and is enriched densely with nerve endings.[81,82] The clitoris is stabilized during intercourse by the suspensory ligament that connects it to both the mons and symphysis pubis.[83] The glans is also connected to the vestibular bulbs by thin erectile tissues (i.e., similar erectile tissues also surround the lower third of the urethra connecting it to the bulbs and making it homologous to the male corpus spongiosum).[67,76] Clitoral index is an important measure of virilization, is calculated as the product of length and width of the glans, and is considered abnormal if more than 35 mm^2.[82,84]

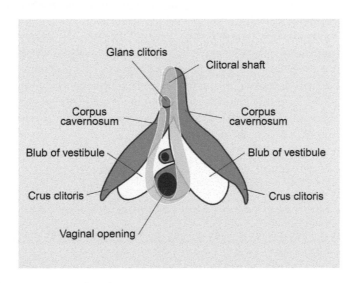

FIG. 1.13

Illustration of clitoral general anatomy.

Original images at Shutterstock, by Denissenko Oleg and is available at https://www.shutterstock.com/ image-vector/structure-clitoris-medical-poster-female-anatomy-1197679213.

Lying between both labia minora is a cavity (the vestibule) that contains the openings of the vagina, the urethra, the Bartholin's glands, and the lesser vestibular glands.[67] Sexual arousal leads to its congestion and it protects the urethra like an air bag during intercourse (i.e., the lack of such protection—for whatever etiology—can cause recurrent and postcoital cystitis).[66] Vestibular bulbs (aka clitoral bulbs) are two 3-cm-long erectile bodies that lie lateral to the vaginal opening under the skin of the labia minora and extend from the base of the glans clitoris, where they meet anterior to the vaginal and the urethral openings as pars intermedia, to both great vestibular glands (i.e., that are homologous to the male bulbourethral glands and secrete mucous during sexual arousal) posteriorly with their expanded ends; they also contact the perineal membrane inferiorly and are superficially covered by the bulbospongiosus muscle at their posterior aspect.[67,76] At about 2.5 cm below the clitoris and above the vaginal orifice, the urethra opens through a distensible meatus that can have various shapes (i.e., slit-like, rounded, or crescentic); Skene's glands (aka paraurethral glands) open laterally on each side of the urethral opening (i.e., they provide secretions during arousal as well).[66,67]

As for the vascular supply, the superficial and deep external pudendal branches of the femoral artery supply the superior portion of the vulva while the internal pudendal artery supplies the inferior portion.[67] The skin of the vulva drains into the external pudendal vein and then into the long saphenous vein while the clitoris drains into both the deep and superficial dorsal veins and then into the pudendal (internal and external) and long saphenous veins.[67] Lymphatic drainage of clitoris pours directly into the deep inguinal nodes (i.e., and sometimes directly into the internal iliac nodes), that of the lower labia majora pours into the rectal plexus, and that coming collectively from the vulval skin pours into the superficial inguinal nodes, then into the deep ones, and finally into the pelvic nodes.[67] The nervous supply of the vulva mainly comes from the pudendal nerve (S2, S3, and S4) that gives off three branches: the inferior rectal nerve, the perineal nerve, and the dorsal nerve of the clitoris; the labia majora receives different innervation that comes from the ilioinguinal nerve (L1) (i.e., for the anterior third), the posterior labial branches of the perineal nerve (S3) (i.e., for the posterior two-thirds), and the perineal branch of the posterior cutaneous nerve of the thigh (S2) (i.e., for the lateral aspect).[74]

References

1. Carlson BM. *Human Embryology and Developmental Biology.* 5th ed. Philadelphia: Elsevier Saunders; 2014.
2. Guo F, Yan L, Guo H, et al. The transcriptome and DNA methylome landscapes of human primordial germ cells. *Cell.* 2015;161(6):1437–1452.
3. Arboleda VA, Quigley CA, Vilain E. Chapter 118—Genetic basis of gonadal and genital development. In: Jameson JL, De Groot LJ, de Kretser DM, et al., eds. *Endocrinology: Adult and Pediatric.* vol. II. 7th ed. Philadelphia: Elsevier Saunders; 2016.
4. Nicol B, Grimm SA, Chalmel F, et al. RUNX1 maintains the identity of the fetal ovary through an interplay with FOXL2. *Nat Commun.* 2019;10(1):5116.

5. Uhlenhaut NH, Jakob S, Anlag K, et al. Somatic sex reprogramming of adult ovaries to testes by FOXL2 ablation. *Cell.* 2009;139(6):1130–1142.

6. Ohinata Y, Payer B, O'Carroll D, et al. Blimp1 is a critical determinant of the germ cell lineage in mice. *Nature.* 2005;436(7048):207–213.

7. Motta PM, Makabe S, Nottola SA. The ultrastructure of human reproduction. I. The natural history of the female germ cell: origin, migration and differentiation inside the developing ovary. *Hum Reprod Update.* 1997;3(3):281–295.

8. Strauss III JF, Williams CJ. Chapter 8: Ovarian life cycle. In: Strauss JF, Barbieri RL, Gargiulo AR, eds. *Yen & Jaffe's Reproductive Endocrinology: Physiology, Pathophysiology, and Clinical Management.* vol. 1. 8th ed. Philadelphia: Elsevier; 2019.

9. Aramaki S, Hayashi K, Kurimoto K, et al. A mesodermal factor, T, specifies mouse germ cell fate by directly activating germline determinants. *Dev Cell.* 2013;27(5):516–529.

10. Rodriguez A, Matzuk MM, Pangas SA, Strauss JF, Barbieri RL, Gargiulo AR. Chapter 6: Growth factors and reproduction. In: *Yen & Jaffe's Reproductive Endocrinology: Physiology, Pathophysiology, and Clinical Management.* vol. 1. 8th ed. Philadelphia: Elsevier; 2019.

11. Mollgard K, Jespersen A, Lutterodt MC, Yding Andersen C, Hoyer PE, Byskov AG. Human primordial germ cells migrate along nerve fibers and Schwann cells from the dorsal hind gut mesentery to the gonadal ridge. *Mol Hum Reprod.* 2010;16(9):621–631.

12. Chawengsaksophak K, Svingen T, Ng ET, et al. Loss of Wnt5a disrupts primordial germ cell migration and male sexual development in mice. *Biol Reprod.* 2012;86(1):1–12.

13. Tanaka SS, Yamaguchi YL, Steiner KA, et al. Loss of Lhx1 activity impacts on the localization of primordial germ cells in the mouse. *Dev Dyn.* 2010;239(11):2851–2859.

14. Molyneaux KA, Zinszner H, Kunwar PS, et al. The chemokine SDF1/CXCL12 and its receptor CXCR4 regulate mouse germ cell migration and survival. *Development.* 2003;130(18):4279–4286.

15. Chuva SM, van de Driesche S, Carvalho RLC, et al. Altered primordial germ cell migration in the absence of transforming growth factor B signaling via ALK5. *Dev Biol.* 2005;284(1):194–203.

16. Morohashi K. The ontogenesis of the steroidogenic tissues. *Genes Cells.* 1997;2(2):95–106.

17. Capel B. The battle of the sexes. *Mech Dev.* 2000;92(1):89–103.

18. Moore KL. *The Developing Human: Clinically Oriented Embryology.* 10th ed. Philadelphia: Elsevier; 2016.

19. Birk OS, Casiano DE, Wassif CA, et al. The LIM homeobox gene Lhx9 is essential for mouse gonad formation. *Nature.* 2000;403(6772):909–913.

20. Hu YC, Okumura LM, Page DC. Gata4 is required for formation of the genital ridge in mice. *PLoS Genet.* 2013;9(7), e1003629.

21. Cotinot C, Pailhoux E, Jaubert F, Fellous M. Molecular genetics of sex determination. *Semin Reprod Med.* 2002;20(3):157–167.

22. Kohler B, Lin L, Ferraz-de-Souza B, et al. Five novel mutations in steroidogenic factor 1 (SF1, NR5A1) in 46,XY patients with severe underandrogenization but without adrenal insufficiency. *Hum Mutat.* 2008;29(1):59–64.

23. Bulun SE. Chapter 17: Physiology and pathology of the female reproductive axis. In: Melmed S, Polonsky KS, Larsen PR, Kronenberg HM, eds. *Williams Textbook of Endocrinology.* 13th ed. Philadelphia: Elsevier; 2016.

24. Warr N, Greenfield A. The molecular and cellular basis of gonadal sex reversal in mice and humans. *Wiley Interdiscip Rev Dev Biol.* 2012;1(4):559–577.

25. Kumar S, Chatzi C, Brade T, Cunningham TJ, Zhao X, Duester G. Sex-specific timing of meiotic initiation is regulated by Cyp26b1 independent of retinoic acid signalling. *Nat Commun.* 2011;2(1):1–8.
26. Wang HU, Chen ZF, Anderson DJ. Molecular distinction and Angiogenic interaction between embryonic arteries and veins revealed by ephrin-B2 and its receptor Eph-B4. *Cell.* 1998;93(5):741–753.
27. Capel B, Albercht KH, Washburn LL, Eicher EM. Migration of mesonephric cells into the mammalian gonad depends on Sry. *Mech Dev.* 1999;84(1–2):127–131.
28. Bardoni B, Zanaria E, Guioli S, et al. A dosage sensitive locus at chromosome Xp21 is involved in male to female sex reversal. *Nat Genet.* 1994;7(4):497–501.
29. Meeks JJ, Crawford SE, Russell TA, Morohashi KI, Weiss J, Jameson JL. Dax1 regulates testis cord organization during gonadal differentiation. *Development.* 2003;130(5):1029–1036.
30. Ludbrook LM, Harley VR. Sex determination: a 'window' of DAX1 activity. *Trends Endocrinol Metab.* 2004;15(3):116–121.
31. Coveney D, Cool J, Oliver T, Capel B. Four-dimensional analysis of vascularization during primary development of an organ, the gonad. *Proc Natl Acad Sci USA.* 2008;105(20):7212–7217.
32. Hughes IA, Acerini CL. Factors controlling testis descent. *Eur J Endocrinol.* 2008;159(Suppl. 1):S75–S82.
33. Matsumoto AM, Bremner WJ. Testicular disorders. In: Melmed S, Polonsky KS, Larsen PR, Kronenberg HM, eds. *Williams Textbook of Endocrinology.* 13th ed. Philadelphia: Elsevier; 2016.
34. Adham IM, Agoulnik AI. Insulin-like 3 signalling in testicular descent. *Int J Androl.* 2004;27(5):257–265.
35. Foresta C, Zuccarello D, Garolla A, Ferlin A. Role of hormones, genes, and environment in human cryptorchidism. *Endocr Rev.* 2008;29(5):560–580.
36. Rey R, Picard JY. Embryology and endocrinology of genital development. *Baillieres Clin Endocrinol Metab.* 1998;12(1):17–33.
37. Tong SYC, Huston JM, Watts LM. Does testosterone diffuse down the Wolffian duct during sexual differentiation? *J Urol.* 1996;155(6):2057–2059.
38. Warne GL, Kanumakala S. Molecular endocrinology of sex differentiation. *Semin Reprod Med.* 2002;20(3):169–180.
39. Heikkila M, Peltoketo H, Vainio S. Wnts and the female reproductive system. *J Exp Zool A Ecol Genet Physiol.* 2001;290(6):616–623.
40. Dolle P, Izpisua-Belmonte JC, Brown JM, Tickle C, Duboule D. HOX-4 genes and the morphogenesis of mammalian genitalia. *Genes Dev.* 1991;5(10):1767–1776.
41. Goodman FR, Bacchelli C, Brady AF, et al. Novel HOXA13 mutations and the phenotypic spectrum of hand-foot-genital syndrome. *Am J Hum Genet.* 2000;67(1):197–202.
42. Achermann JC, Weiss J, Lee EJ, Jameson JL. Inherited disorders of the gonadotropin hormones. *Mol Cell Endocrinol.* 2001;179(1–2):89–96.
43. Svechnikov K, Landreh L, Weisser J, et al. Origin, development and regulation of human Leydig cells. *Horm Res Paediatr.* 2010;73(2):93–101.
44. de Kretser DM, Loveland K, O'Bryan M. Chapter 136—Spermatogenesis. In: Jameson JL, De Groot LJ, de Kretser DM, et al., eds. *Endocrinology: Adult and Pediatric.* vol. II. 7th ed. Philadelphia: Elsevier Saunders; 2016.
45. Lubs HA. Testicular size in Klinefelter's syndrome in men over fifty: report of a case with XXY/XY mosaicism. *NEJM.* 1962;267(7):326–331.

46. Tishler PV. Diameter of testicles. *NEJM*. 1971;285(26):1489.

47. Sotos JF, Tokar NJ. Appraisal of testicular volumes: volumes matching ultrasound values referenced to stages of genital development [published correction appears in Int J Pediatr Endocrinol. 2017;2017:10]. *Int J Pediatr Endocrinol*. 2017;2017(7):1–10. https://doi.org/10.1186/s13633-017-0046-x.

48. Jaiswal VK, Khadilkar V, Khadilkar A, Lohiya N. Stretched penile length and testicular size from birth to 18 years in boys. *Indian J Endocrinol Metab*. 2019;23(1):3–8.

49. Standring S, Anand N, Birch R, et al. Chapter 76: Male reproductive system. In: Standring S, ed. *Gray's Anatomy: The Anatomical Basis of Clinical Practice*. 41st ed. New York: Elsevier Limited; 2016.

50. Wang YN, Zeng Q, Xiong F, Zeng Y. Male external genitalia growth curves and charts for children and adolescents aged 0 to 17 years in Chongqing, China. *Asian J Androl*. 2018;20(6):567–571.

51. Goede J, Hack WWM, Sijstermans K, et al. Normative values for testicular volume measured by ultrasonography in a normal population from infancy to adolescence. *Horm Res Paediatr*. 2011;76(1):56–64.

52. Barak S, Baker HWG. Chapter 141—Clinical management of male infertility. In: Jameson JL, De Groot LJ, de Kretser DM, et al., eds. *Endocrinology: Adult and Pediatric*. vol. II. 7th ed. Philadelphia: Elsevier Saunders; 2016.

53. Liu PY, Veldhuis JD. Chapter 12: Hypothalamo-pituitary unit, testis, and male accessory organs. In: Strauss JF, Barbieri RL, Gargiulo AR, eds. *Yen & Jaffe's Reproductive Endocrinology: Physiology, Pathophysiology, and Clinical Management*. vol. 1. 8th ed. Philadelphia: Elsevier; 2019.

54. Amann RP, Howards SS. Daily spermatozoal production and epididymal spermatozoal reserves of the human male. *J Urol*. 1980;124(2):211–215.

55. Clermont Y. Kinetics of spermatogenesis in mammals: seminiferous epithelium cycle and spermatogonial renewal. *Physiol Rev*. 1972;52(1):198–236.

56. Harrison RG, Barclay AE. The distribution of the testicular artery (internal spermatic artery) to the human testis. *Br J Urol*. 1948;20(2):57–66.

57. Raman JD, Goldstein M. Intraoperative characterization of arterial vasculature in spermatic cord. *Urology*. 2004;64(3):561–564.

58. Zini A, Boman JM. Varicocele: red flag or red herring? *Semin Reprod Med*. 2009;27(2):171–178.

59. Taguchi K, Tsukamoto T, Murakami G. Anatomical studies of the autonomic nervous system in the human pelvis by the whole-mount staining method: left-right communicating nerves between bilateral pelvic plexuses. *J Urol*. 1999;161(1):320–325.

60. Kraft KH, Mucksavage P, Canning DA, Snyder III HM, Kolon TF. Histological findings in patients with cryptorchidism and testis-epididymis nonfusion. *J Urol*. 2011;186(5):2045–2049.

61. Clement P, Giuliano F. Anatomy and physiology of genital organs—men. *Handb Clin Neurol*. 2015;130(3rd series):19–37.

62. Turner TT, D'Addario D, Howards SS. Further observations on the initiation of sperm motility. *Biol Reprod*. 1978;19(5):1095–1101.

63. Rowley MJ, Teshima F, Heller CG. Duration of transit of spermatozoa through the human male ductular system. *Obstet Gynecol Surv*. 1971;26(1):390–396.

64. Hoffer AP. The ultrastructure of the ductus deferens in man. *Biol Reprod*. 1976;14(4):425–443.

65. Anawalt BD, Braunstein GD. Testes. In: Gardner DG, Shoback D, eds. *Greenspan's Basic & Clinical Endocrinology*. 10th ed. New York: McGraw Hill Education; 2018.

66. Graziottin A, Gambini D. Anatomy and physiology of genital organs—women. *Handb Clin Neurol.* 2015;130(3rd series):39–60.

67. Standring S, Anand N, Birch R, et al. *Gray's Anatomy: The Anatomical Basis of Clinical Practice.* 41st ed. New York: Elsevier Limited; 2016.

68. Conti M, Chang RJ. Chapter 125—Folliculogenesis, ovulation, and luteogenesis. In: Jameson JL, De Groot LJ, de Kretser DM, et al., eds. *Endocrinology: Adult and Pediatric.* vol. II. 7th ed. Philadelphia: Elsevier Saunders; 2016.

69. Bardo DME, Black M, Schenk K, et al. Location of the ovaries in girls from newborn to 18 years of age: reconsidering ovarian shielding. *Yearbook Diagn Radiol.* 2010;2010(2010):169–170.

70. Erickson GF, Magoffin DA, Dyer CA, Hofeditz C. The ovarian androgen producing cells: a review of structure/function relationships. *Endocr Rev.* 1985;6(3):371–399.

71. Lee JF, Mauror VM, Block GE. Anatomic relations of pelvic autonomic nerves to pelvic operations. *Arch Surg.* 1973;107(2):324–328.

72. Kurita T. Normal and abnormal epithelial differentiation in the female reproductive tract. *Differentiation.* 2011;82(3):117–126.

73. Minto CL, Hollings N, Hall-Craggs M, Creighton S. Magnetic resonance imaging in the assessment of complex Müllerian anomalies. *Br J Obstet Gynaecol.* 2001;108(8):791–797.

74. Shoja MM, Sharma A, Mirzayan N, et al. Neuroanatomy of the female abdominopelvic region: a review with application to pelvic pain syndromes. *Clin Anat.* 2013;26(1):66–76.

75. Chen C, Huang L, Liu P, et al. Neurovascular quantitative study of the uterosacral ligament related to nerve-sparing radical hysterectomy. *Eur J Obstet Gynecol Reprod Biol.* 2014;172(2014):74–79.

76. O'Connell HE, DeLancey JO. Clitoral anatomy in nulliparous, healthy, premenopausal volunteers using unenhanced magnetic resonance imaging. *J Urol.* 2005;173(6):2060–2063.

77. Kimberley N, Huston JM, Southwell BR, Grover SR. Vaginal agenesis, the hymen, and associated anomalies. *J Pediatr Adolesc Gynecol.* 2012;25(1):54–58.

78. Yavagal S, de Farias T, Medina C, Takacs P. Normal vulvovaginal, perineal, and pelvic anatomy with reconstructive considerations. *Semin Plast Surg.* 2011;25(2):121–129.

79. Ostrzenski A. G-spot anatomy and its clinical significance: a systematic review. *Clin Anat.* 2019;32(8):1094–1101.

80. Jannini EA, Whipple B, Kingsberg SA, Buisson O, Foldes P, Vardi Y. Who's afraid of the G-spot? *J Sex Med.* 2010;7(1):25–34.

81. Yang CC, Cold CJ, Yilmaz U, Maravilla KR. Sexually responsive vascular tissue of the vulva. *BJU Int.* 2006;97(4):766–772.

82. Verkauf BS, Von Thron J, O'Brien WF. Clitoral size in normal women. *Obstet Gynecol.* 1992;80(1):41–44.

83. Rees MA, O'Connell HE, Plenter RJ, Huston JM. The suspensory ligament of the clitoris: connective tissue supports of the erectile tissues of the female urogenital region. *Clin Anat.* 2000;13(6):397–403.

84. Tagatz GE, Kopher RA, Nagel TC, Okagaki T. The clitoral index: a bioassay of androgenic stimulation. *Obstet Gynecol.* 1979;54(5):562–564.

Reproductive endocrine physiology

2

Sairabanu Sokwala (Mohamed Rashid)

Diabetes Care Centre, MP Shah Hospital, Nairobi, Kenya

Chapter outline

Subfertility. https://doi.org/10.1016/B978-0-323-75945-8.00002-5

Physiology of the male reproductive system
Introduction

The male reproductive physiology involves external structures (scrotum and penis) and internal structures (testis, epididymis, vas deferens, and prostate). These are well vascularized and supported by several other glands. The primary male androgen hormone is testosterone produced by Leydig cells in the testis, but other hormones like inhibin and Mullerian-inhibiting substance produced by Sertoli cells also contribute to the male reproductive physiology. Follicular-stimulating hormone (FSH) and luteinizing hormone (LH), produced from the anterior pituitary, under control of the hypothalamic hormone, gonadotropin-releasing hormone (GnRH) are involved in the regulation of the male reproductive physiology and together these hormones form the hypothalamic–pituitary–gonadal axis.

Functions of male reproductive organs

The male reproductive system, through the hypothalamic–pituitary–gonadal axis, is responsible for male sexual development/maturity, including the formation of secondary sex characteristics for males. In addition, it is necessary for sperm production (spermatogenesis) and lifelong maintenance of male sexuality. The male reproductive system also assists in the transport of generated sperms into the female reproductive system for fertilization. Sperm production and transport occur in the testis, alongside the production of the male androgen, testosterone. Thus, the testes have exocrine and endocrine functions simultaneously.[1]

Internal male reproductive organs

a. **Testes:** Paired male sex organs located in the scrotum, normally 4–5 cm in size, these are the sites for spermatogenesis and male sex hormone production (Fig. 2.1). Each testis consists of 300–400 lobules, consisting of seminiferous tubules. Spermatogenesis occurs within the lining of the lumen of these tubules. Inside the seminiferous tubules are two main types of cells, Sertoli/supporting cells and germ cells[1]:

   i. *Sertoli cells:* These are long and branching supportive cells, located on the basement membrane of seminiferous tubules, extending toward the lumen and surround the germ cells. They produce molecules that assist in signaling to promote spermatogenesis and determine the survival of sperm cells. They have a crucial role in forming the blood–testis barrier through tight junctions between them; this, in turn, is important to keep blood infections/substances away from germ cells and to prevent antigens on germ cells from entering the bloodstream. This could otherwise evoke an autoimmune response.

   ii. *Germ cells:* There are at least 13 different types of germ cells, each representing a specific process in spermatogenesis. These include dark type A spermatogonia

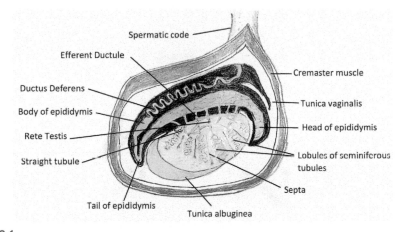

FIG. 2.1

Functional anatomy and sperm transport structure in the testis.

(Ad), pale type A spermatogonia (Ap), type B spermatogonia (B), preleptotene (R), leptotene (L), zygotene (Z), pachytene primary spermatocytes (P), secondary spermatocytes (II), spermatids (Sa, Sb, Sc, Sd), and sperms.[1]

Leydig cells, located in the interstitium of the testis, between the seminiferous tubules, produce testosterone.

Spermatogenesis

This is the process of sperm production, beginning at puberty and continues throughout a man's life, occurring in cycles of about 64 days (ranges from 42 to 76 days), with cycles beginning about every 16 days. There is no synchrony between different sections of the seminiferous tubules, though.[2]

Spermatogenesis occurs through three phases (Fig. 2.2):

1. **Proliferation phase:** This involves the division of spermatogonia for either self-renewal or differentiation into daughter cells that will become mature gametes. It comprises a single cell division resulting in two identical diploid daughter cells (type B spermatogonia to primary spermatocyte). Type B spermatogonia are derived by the division of pale type A spermatogonia in the basal, stem cell niche of seminiferous tubules. One of type B spermatogonia remains a spermatogonium to undergo further mitosis, the other proceeds to meiotic phase. Cytoplasm between the spermatogonial cells forms connections between cells, which persist throughout spermatogenesis and are thought to be crucial for cellular development and gene expression.[2]

2. **Meiotic phase:** This is the phase of division, with the reduction of germ cells to haploid spermatids with half the DNA. Unlike mitosis where two diploid genetically identical daughter cells are formed, in meiosis, four haploid genetically diverse daughter cells are formed. This involves two steps: primary spermatocyte to secondary spermatocyte and secondary spermatocyte to Sa spermatid.

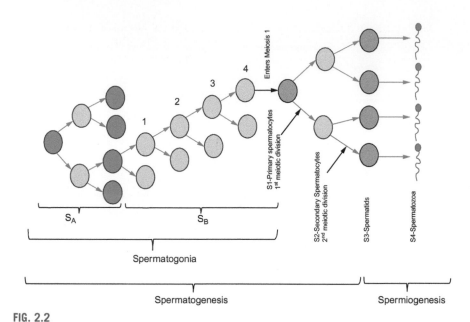

FIG. 2.2

Spermatogenesis and spermiogenesis.

3. **Spermiogenesis phase:** Sa spermatids change to mature spermatozoa through nucleus and cytoplasmic modifications including cytoplasmic loss, organelle migration, acrosome formation, flagellum formation from a centriole, nuclear compression leading to asymmetrical shape and mitochondrial restructuring. These changes are assisted by various cellular elements. When spermatid elongation is complete, Sertoli cell cytoplasm is pulled back, thus removing excess cytoplasm and pushing the developed sperm into the tubular lumen. Almost 300 sperms per gram of testis per second are produced.[2]

Structure of formed sperm

The volume of the sperm is 85,000 times less than an ovum, and daily about 100–300 million sperms are produced. A mature sperm consists of the head, containing minimal cytoplasm, a compact nucleus and the acrosome "cap" with lysosomal enzymes that aid the penetration of the ovum; mid-piece containing mitochondria for ATP production that is necessary for flagella movement; tail, which mainly contains the flagella (Fig. 2.3).[2]

Sperm storage and transport

For its final function of fertilization of an ovum, the sperm needs to move from the seminiferous tubules in the testis, through the epididymis and via the penis during ejaculation, to the female genital tract.[1,2]

- *Role of epididymis:* Approximately 6 m long, the epididymis is a coiled structure, where sperm transport, fertilizing capacity, motility maturation, and storage occur. Immotile sperms enter the epididymis head (caput epididymis) with testicular fluid and are moved along the coils by contraction of muscles lining the epididymal tubes (corpus epididymis) as they mature into motile sperms. The most mature sperms, ready for fertilization (both binding and penetration), are stored in the tail end of the epididymis (cauda epididymis), to be released during ejaculation. This transit takes about 2–12 days.
- *Duct systems and ejaculation:* Mature sperms leave the epididymis during ejaculation, to enter the ductus/vas deferens. Ductus deferens passes through the inguinal canal posteriorly to the pelvic cavity, terminating in a dilated ampulla posterior to the bladder.
- *Accessory glands and functions:* sperms contribute about 5% of the semen volume, most of which is provided by fluid from the accessory glands as detailed as follows:
  - *Seminal vesicles:* The ampulla of ductus deferens opens into the ejaculatory duct, which also receives fluid from seminal vesicles, paired glands that produce fructose-rich fluid contributing up to 60% of semen volume and necessary for ATP production. This fluid and sperm combination moves next to the prostate through the paired ejaculatory ducts.
  - *Prostate gland:* When seminal fluid passes through the prostate, an alkaline milky fluid is added, which temporarily coagulates the semen, a step necessary to retain sperm in the female reproductive system to allow fructose consumption for motility. The prostate fluid then aids in decoagulation, to allow fluidity of semen for further transit.
  - *Bulbourethral/Cowper's glands:* Fluid from these glands is added just before semen release and is thick and salty, helping in the lubrication of female external genitalia and clearing urethral urine residues.

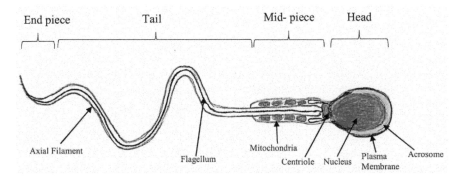

End piece   Tail   Mid-piece   Head

Axial Filament

Flagellum

Mitochondria

Centriole   Nucleus

Plasma Membrane

Acrosome

FIG. 2.3

Structure of spermatozoa.

Physiology of male sexual response

There are four stages of male sexual response: excitement, plateau, orgasm, and resolution. The initial event is erection, followed by orgasm and then ejaculation as detailed as follows:

Penile erection: This results from various neurovascular, molecular, psychological, and endocrinological factors. It is initiated by visual, olfactory, or imaginative stimuli in the medial preoptic area and paraventricular nucleus in the hypothalamus and involves dopamine, norepinephrine, oxytocin, nitric oxide (NO), α-melanocyte-stimulating hormone, and opioid peptides. Tactile genital stimulation mediates penile tumescence through parasympathetic sacral reflex arc, whereas psychogenic tumescence mainly involves central suppression of sympathetic stimulation.[3] Neuronal and endothelial NO synthases increase NO levels during initiation and maintenance of erection, respectively, causing vasodilatation and smooth muscle relaxation, thus increasing blood flow to the penis with reduced venous return.

Orgasm: This is the period preceding ejaculation after penile erection, which involves hyperventilation, tachycardia, high blood pressure, pelvic muscle and rectal sphincter contractions, and facial grimacing.[4]

Ejaculation: It involves the emission of semen into the urethra and expulsion out of the urethra. Emission is mediated by sympathetic nerves in the pelvic plexus, eliciting contraction of smooth muscles in vas deferens, seminal vesicles, and prostate and has a central cerebral control,[5] whereas expulsion is mediated by efferent pathways in pudendal nerves through the contractions of striated muscles (bulbospongiosus and ischiocavernosus).[6]

Male sex hormones and functions

Male sex hormones, termed "androgens," include testosterone, the primary male sex hormone, dihydrotestosterone (DHT), and androstenedione.

Testosterone

Testosterone is secreted from the interstitial cells of Leydig, which are in large concentration in the testis in newborns and adult males after puberty. About 97% of testosterone gets bound to plasma albumin or sex-hormone-binding globulin and circulates to the tissues, where most of the testosterone is converted to DHT, particularly in male fetus (for development of external genitalia) and adult prostate. Unused testosterone is converted in the liver to androsterone and dehydroepiandrosterone (DHEA) and conjugated as glucuronides or sulfates, which are excreted by the gut or kidney. The biosynthesis of testosterone is summarized in Fig. 2.4A.

Mechanism of action: Testosterone is converted to DHT by cytoplasmic 5α-reductase. DHT combined with a receptor protein, enters the nucleus, and binds to nuclear proteins, where it induces DNA–RNA transcription, increasing cellular protein production and increased cell numbers.

Functions of testosterone: These have been detailed in Table 2.1. In general, testosterone is mainly responsible for specific male masculine characteristics. During

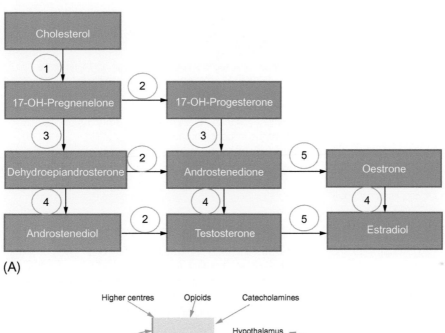

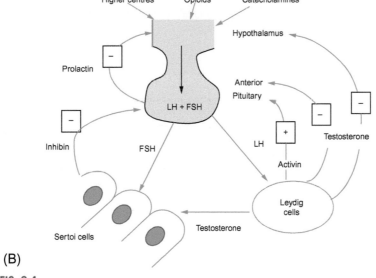

FIG. 2.4

(A) Testosterone biosynthesis pathway: (1) desmolase; (2) 3β-hydroxysteroid dehydrogenase; (3) 17,20-desmolase; (4) 17β-hydroxysteroid dehydrogenase; and (5) aromatase. (B) Hypothalamic–pituitary–testis axis in males. +, positive feedback; −, negative feedback; FSH, follicular-stimulating hormone; LH, luteinizing hormone; GnRH, gonadotropin-releasing hormone.

Table 2.1 Functions of testosterone in males.[7]

Function	Description
Fetal male development	Testosterone secreted by genital ridge and fetal testis stimulates the formation of penis, scrotum, prostate, seminal vesicles, and male genital ducts. It suppresses female genital organ formation
Descent of testis	Testis descend in scrotum in last 2–3 months of gestation under the influence of testosterone
Development of adult primary sexual characteristics	After puberty, testosterone causes penile, scrotal, and testicular enlargement
Development of adult secondary sexual characteristics: these include:	
- Distribution of body hair	Testosterone causes male-pattern hair distribution over the pubis, along linea alba, face, chest, and back
- Male-pattern baldness	Testosterone decreases hair growth on top of the head
- Male voice	Testosterone stimulates laryngeal enlargement and hypertrophy of laryngeal mucosa, leading to male voice
- Increased skin thickness	Testosterone contributes to ruggedness in male skin and increases secretion from sebaceous glands
- Protein formation and muscle development	Testosterone stimulates protein synthesis and deposition alongside increasing muscle mass
- Increased bone matrix and calcium retention	Due to protein anabolic effect, testosterone increases overall bone matrix and thus calcium salt retention. Testosterone also increases epiphyseal union. Effects on pelvis include lengthening, narrowing, giving it funnel-like shape, and strengthening for load bearing
- Increased basal metabolic rate	Increased testosterone levels during early adulthood contribute to 5%–10% increased metabolic rate, possibly due to protein anabolic effect by increased enzyme formation
- Increased red blood cells	Males have 700,000 more red blood cells vs women, possibly due to increased metabolic rate
- Effect on water and electrolyte balance	Testosterone has a small effect on increasing sodium reabsorption at distal renal tubules. During puberty, this could contribute to increased weight due to blood and extracellular fluid volume expansion by 5%–10%

early fetal life (first trimester), chorionic gonadotropin stimulates testosterone production, to adult levels. This is to enable masculine genital tract differentiation. In infant boys, serum testosterone (T) concentrations that are gonadal in origin increase to pubertal concentrations between 1 and 3 months of age and fall to prepubertal values around 6 months of age, and this is of undetermined significance. After this surge, testosterone production stops through infantile age, due to tonically suppressed

GnRH production; this is then followed by another surge at ages 10–13 years, when anterior pituitary gonadotropic hormones stimulate its production at puberty onset, in response to the intermittent GnRH production. This production continues till age 50 years where production reduces gradually.[8,9]

Interplay of endocrine and reproductive systems

The male reproductive system is controlled by GnRH from the arcuate nucleus of hypothalamus, which is released in a pulsatile manner every 1–3 h, and transported through the hypophysio-pituitary portal system to the anterior pituitary where it stimulates gonadotrope cells to release gonadotropins: FSH and LH. LH production is more pulsatile than FSH and both gonadotropins work by stimulating cAMP second messenger systems (Fig. 2.4B).

FSH stimulates spermatogenesis by its action on Sertoli cells in seminiferous tubules, whereas LH stimulates testicular Leydig cells to produce testosterone. Both FSH and testosterone are needed for spermatogenesis.

Testosterone production provides a negative feedback to the hypothalamus to reduce GnRH production and to the pituitary to reduce LH production. Thus, both FSH and LH productions are regulated by circulating testosterone levels.[9]

Inhibin, a glycoprotein produced by Sertoli cells when spermatogenesis proceeds increasingly, plays a role in inhibiting FSH release, thus regulating spermatogenesis.[9]

Puberty

Puberty is a transition period from childhood to adulthood and involves physiologic, constitutional, and somatic changes associated with changes in external and internal genitalia and secondary sex characteristics.[10] Puberty begins when GnRH secretion breaks through the childhood inhibition by sex hormones, for unknown reasons, causing increased gonadotropins and downstream changes including gonadal development and maturation, sex steroid hormone release, and gamete development.[11] Pulsatile GnRH secretion is mediated by "GnRH pulse generators" in the hypothalamus, mainly due to neuropeptides: KNDy-kisspeptins, neurokinin-B (NKB), and dynorphin (Dyn).[12]

Leptin has a key role in pubertal development by suppressing neuropeptide Y, which suppresses GnRH release.

Puberty in males

Pituitary LH stimulates testosterone production (as mentioned earlier), which stimulates secondary sex characteristics formation, alongside control of LH secretion, whereas FSH, controlled by Sertoli cell released inhibin, stimulates spermatogenesis. Sex hormone-binding globulin levels also reduce with the onset of puberty. Tanner stages of pubertal development are summarized in Table 2.2.[13]

Table 2.2 Tanner stages of pubertal development in boys and girls.[13]

Physical development (boys)		Physical development (girls)	
Stage	**Description**	**Stage**	**Description**
G1	Prepubertal—testis volume <3 mL	B1	No palpable breast tissue, but papilla elevation—prepubertal
PH1	No pubic hair	PH1	No pubic hair
G2	Testis volume 3–6 mL. Minimal penile change	B2	Small mound of breast budding with breast and papilla elevation
PH2	Soft, light pubic hair	PH2	Soft, light pubic hair
G3	Testis volume 8–12 mL. Lengthening of penis	B3	Enlargement of breast and areola
PH3	Darker curled, and rougher hair	PH3	Darker curled, and rougher hair
G4	Testis volume 12–15 mL. Lengthening and broadening of penis	G4	Areola and papilla project, forming "double mound" above the breast level
PH4	Terminal hair over pubic triangle plus external genitalia but not the thighs	PH4	Terminal hair over pubic triangle plus external genitalia but not the thighs Menarche between 4th and 5th stages
G5	Testis volume >15 mL. Adult genital organs	B5	Breasts are mature adult size/shape with alveolar recession to breast-level papillary projection and loss of double mound
PH5	Terminal hair extending to medial aspect of thighs	PH5	Terminal hair extends to medial aspect of thighs

B, breast development; G, genital development; PH, pubic hair development.

Physiology of the female reproductive system
Introduction

The female reproductive system is mostly located internally rather than externally unlike its male counterpart. It functions not only to produce hormones and gametes, but also to maintain a pregnancy to term and delivery of the fetus. External female genitalia (vulva) include vagina, mons pubis, labia majora, labia minora, clitoris, urethra, vulva vestibule, vestibular bulbs, Skene's glands, and Bartholin's glands, whereas internal female genitalia comprise the ovaries, fallopian tubes, uterus, and cervix. Control of the female reproductive system is by the hypothalamic–pituitary–ovarian system with close interactions between hormonal, metabolic–energetic, genetic–epigenetic, and intra- and extraovarian factors.

The female reproductive physiology culminating in ovulation and fertility can be viewed as a triple-act theater consisting of prenatal development of ovaries and germ cells as the first act, onset of reproductive maturity (puberty) as the second act, and final act of folliculogenesis, the ovarian cycle and menarche.[14]

Functions of female reproductive organs

The functions of each structure of the female reproductive system are detailed as follows (Fig. 2.5):

External genitalia

a. **Mons pubis:** It forms a cushion during sexual intercourse and secretes pheromones from sebaceous glands for sexual stimulation.[15]
b. **Labia majora and minora:** These function to cover the other external genital structures and get engorged during sexual arousal.
c. **Clitoris:** This is the female sensory sex organ, consisting of about 8000 nerve endings, and becomes erected during sexual arousal.
d. **Vestibular bulbs:** These are sensory organs close to the clitoris and get engorged with blood during sexual arousal, exerting pressure on the clitoris, thus providing an enjoyable feeling during sexual arousal.
e. **Vulva vestibule:** This area between labia minora constitutes the opening to the vagina and urethra.
f. **Bartholin's glands:** Located on each side of the vaginal opening, Bartholin's glands lubricate the vulva and prevent friction during intercourse by secreting a mucus-like substance into the vagina.
g. **Skene's glands:** Located on each side of the urethra, these glands produce a substance, also thought to be the female ejaculate, which has antimicrobial properties to prevent urinary tract infections.

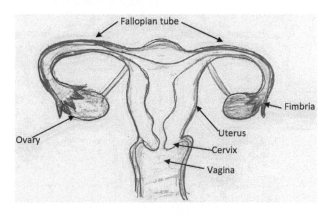

FIG. 2.5

Gross anatomy of the female reproductive system.

h. *Vagina:* The vagina functions as a reservoir for semen while the sperm moves into the cervix and up toward the fallopian tubes. It also forms a conduit for childbirth and menses.

Internal structures

a. *Ovaries:* Oocyte development occurs in the stroma, where each oocyte is surrounded by supporting cells, together forming a follicle. Two main functions of the ovary are ovum generation for fertilization and secretion of estrogen and progesterone to prepare the endometrium for implantation.[16]

b. *Fallopian tubes/uterine tubes:* They form conduits for the oocyte from the ovary to the uterus. They contain an inner mucosal layer consisting of cilia, which moves the oocyte toward the uterus. With rising estrogen levels, ovulation occurs (described in detail later) and a secondary oocyte together with granulosa cells is released from the ovary. In addition, this stimulates smooth muscle contractions of the uterine tube and the oocyte/granulosa complex is taken up by the fimbriae of the tubes. Ciliary movement is also increased by high estrogen levels and this propels the oocyte toward the uterus. Fertilization occurs in the ampulla, the mid-region of the tubes, and multiplication follows as the fertilized ovum (zygote) continues to move toward the uterus, where implantation occurs. If fertilization does not occur, the oocyte is shed in the next menstrual cycle.

c. *Uterus and cervix:* The main functions of the muscular uterus include implantation and nourishment of the growing embryo, facilitating the movement of incoming sperms anteriorly toward the uterine tubes, and shedding of uterine lining if no implantation occurs. Under high estrogen levels, cervical mucus secretion thins down to accommodate sperm movement.

The three layers of the uterus include outer perimetrium, providing covering externally; middle myometrium, assisting in menses and labor; and inner endometrium. Endometrium contains the stratum basalis, which is close to myometrium and stratum functionalis, the thicker, lamina propria, and endothelial layer that forms the implantation site after fertilization and sheds during menses if fertilization does not occur. Estrogen during the follicular phase (see in the following) is crucial for thickening of stratum functionalis in preparation for implantation, and this is then maintained by progesterone during the luteal phase. If implantation occurs, corpus luteum continues producing progesterone following signals from the implanted embryo, whereas if implantation does not occur, corpus luteum degrades, thus reducing progesterone and, in turn, thinning the endometrium alongside reducing blood flow by spiral arteries that get constricted with increased prostaglandin levels. This leads to the shedding of endometrium stratum functionalis layer and white blood cells as menses.

Puberty in females

With an increase in GnRH, there is an increase in LH and FSH in prepubertal females. LH is mainly responsible for androgen (primarily testosterone) production during the follicular phase, from follicular theca cells, whereas FSH causes proliferation of follicular granulosa cells, with increased aromatase activity to convert androgens to estradiol and upregulated LH receptors. Estradiol further upregulates FSH receptors on granulosa cells to increase proliferation. Progesterone also rises, and alongside estradiol promotes the formation of secondary sexual characteristics and modulation of FSH/LH secretion from the pituitary. Sex hormone-binding globulin levels dip during puberty.[17]

The ovarian cycle

This is a roughly 28-day cycle in a female's reproductive years, which involves certain changes in oocytes and ovarian follicles. It includes oogenesis and folliculogenesis (Fig. 2.6).

Oogenesis and oocytes

Oogenesis begins in utero and continues throughout a female's reproductive years (Fig. 2.7).

In utero phase: Primordial germ cells arrive at the genital ridge by the 5th week of the development, when they are labeled as oogonia. These multiply by mitosis without atresia and by 6–7 weeks, about 10,000 oogonia exist. By 8 weeks, 600,000 oogonia are present, which then undergo a simultaneous process of mitosis, meiosis, and atresia, to peak at 20 weeks to 6–7 million cells, of which about 60% are primary oocytes and the rest are oogonia. Oogonial mitosis ends by approximately 7th month and atresia peaks by 5th month, after which, by 7th month, oogonial atresia is complete while follicular atresia sets in, to continue throughout reproductive years.[18] At birth, 1–2 million germ cells persist, which are primary oocytes in prophase of the first meiotic division.[19]

Prepuberty and puberty: Germ cell mass reduces further to 300,000–400,000 at the pubertal onset, out of which only about 400 are taken on for ovulation throughout a female's life span. After the first LH surge at puberty, the primary oocytes complete the 1st meiotic division with conversion to secondary oocyte and the formation of 1st polar body.

Ovulation

At ovulation, the secondary oocyte is released into the fallopian tube alongside granulosa cells. The first polar body disintegrates. If fertilization occurs, a second meiotic division occurs in the secondary oocyte, converting it into an ovum, and the 2nd polar body is expelled.[7] The haploid ovum becomes a diploid zygote upon fertilization by a sperm. The cytoplasm and organelles are contributed to the ovum, which ensures nutrition of the zygote prior to implantation (Fig. 2.6).

Ovulation occurs once every 28 days, throughout reproductive years. Toward mid-cycle, estradiol levels rise, which initially suppress FSH release, leading to atresia of most recruited follicles. However, one follicle survives and proceeds to develop into the dominant follicle, which secretes high levels of estrogen. This is followed by rising LH levels and small rise in FSH levels (the LH surge), through a positive

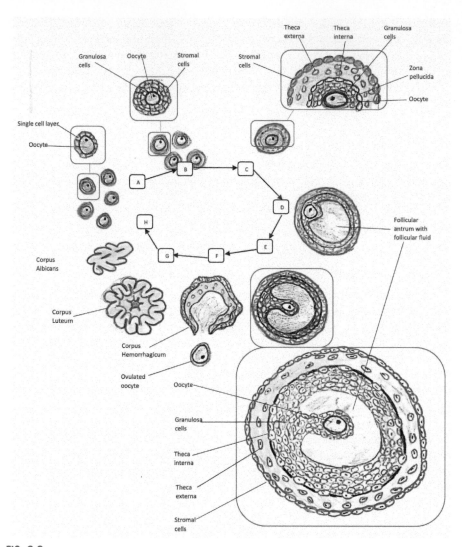

FIG. 2.6

Follicular development and ovulation: A—**The primordial follicle:** single layer of granulosa cells and a single immature oocyte. B—: **double layer of stratified epithelium—zona granulosa** C—**The secondary follicle:** proliferation of granulosa cells and by the final phase of oocyte growth, with theca externa and interna formation. D—**The tertiary follicle:** thecal hypertrophy and appearance of the *antrum*. E—**Graafian follicle:** granulosa cells and oocyte remain encased by the basal lamina. The antral fluid volume increases and when cumulus oophorus forms, Graafian follicle is ready for ovulation. F—Follicular rupture occurs, releasing the oocyte (ovulation) and blood fills the antrum forming **corpus hemorrhagicum.** G—**Corpus luteum:** forms after ovulation and produces steroid hormones. H—Regression of corpus luteum to **corpus albicans.**

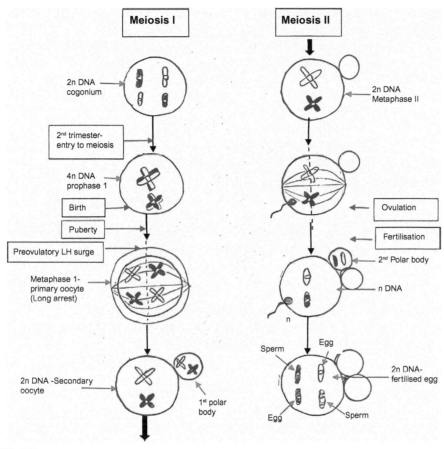

FIG. 2.7

Oogenesis. DNA, deoxyribonucleic acid; n, quantity of DNA material in haploid chromosomes (23).

feedback to the hypothalamus and anterior pituitary. This triggers one dominant follicle to ovulate under LH-mediated prostaglandin release. Ovulation occurs 34–36 h after LH surge, following the rapid enlargement of the dominant follicle, protrusion from the cortical surface as a "stigma" and rupture to release the oocyte cumulus complex into a peritoneal cavity. LH- and HCG-mediated proteases like plasminogen activator contribute to follicular rupture.

Regular ovulation also requires other functional hormones, e.g., thyroid and adrenal hormones; thus, derangements in the levels of these hormones could lead to disruptions in ovulation and contribute to infertility.

Corpus luteum: Restructuring of the dominant follicle, by rapid revascularization and fibroblast migration, occurs after ovulation, forming the corpus luteum (Fig. 2.6). Following this, granulosa and theca cells undergo structural changes termed as luteinization, converting them into granulosa lutein (large) cells and theca-lutein (small) cells, respectively.[20] Under the influence of LH, corpus luteum is the main site for postovulatory steroidogenesis following vascularization with the provision of low-density lipoprotein (LDL) which is taken up by macrophages through steroidogenic acute regulatory protein and thus the production of progesterone.

If pregnancy does not occur, corpus luteum survives for 12–16 days and then regresses by apoptosis to the corpus albicans. During pregnancy, LH and HCG maintain the corpus luteum, which continues producing progesterone till about 6 weeks, when luteoplacental transition occurs, and then, the size decreases gradually till term.[21]

Folliculogenesis

The follicle is the primary functional unit in the ovary, comprising of oocytes and supporting cells, mainly involved in steroidogenesis and germ cell production. There are two types of follicles: nongrowing, constitute 90%–95% of all follicles, and growing, which are divided in four phases—primary, secondary, tertiary, and Graafian follicles (Fig. 2.6). First three phases are regulated by intraovarian mechanisms. Recruitment of follicles for ovulation takes up to 85 days and is FSH-dependent; recruited primordial follicles either mature into Graafian follicles or undergo atresia through apoptosis.[22]

Folliculogenesis begins with the primordial follicle, consisting of primary oocyte surrounded by a monolayer of granulosa cells, some of which after puberty are recruited and activated to transform their granulosa cells from squamous to cuboidal with proliferation. These convert to secondary follicles with further proliferation and addition of connective and vascular tissue with theca cells (for estrogen production). The primary oocyte then secretes the zona pellucida, an acellular membrane necessary for fertilization, alongside the collection of follicular fluid between granulosa cells into an antrum. These follicles are tertiary follicles and the one which persists proceeds for ovulation, where the secondary oocyte is extruded along with a few layers of granulosa cells.

Primordial follicle growth is inhibited by anti-Mullerian hormone (AMH), in the absence of which, rapid depletion of follicles, occurs, as happens with aging. Thus, AMH is a reliable marker for ovarian reserve.[16]

Mural granulosa cells, constituting the outer layer of the developed Graafian follicle preovulation, contain high concentration of gonadotropin receptors and are the main site for steroidogenesis, whereas the granulosa cells surrounding the developing ovum (cumulus oophorus) are involved in the oocyte development.[23]

Theca cell layer: This is a stromal cell layer surrounding granulosa cells in the ovarian follicle, consisting of two layers, theca interna, involved in steroidogenesis by providing C19 precursors to granulosa cells for estrogen production, and theca externa, involved in ovulation.[24]

Female sex hormones and functions

In females, biologically active steroids include estradiol, progesterone, testosterone, and DHT, formed mainly in the ovary, but also in peripheral and target tissues, where substrates like androgen and estrogen precursors are provided by adrenal glands and ovary.

Ovarian steroids

Ovaries secrete C21 steroids: progesterone, pregnenolone, and 17α-hydroxyprogesterone; C19 steroids: dehydroepiandrosterone, androstenedione, and testosterone, which serve as precursors for DHT or estradiol; and C18 steroids: estrogens (Fig. 2.8A).

Estrogens

There are four types of estrogens in females: estrone (E1)—predominant in menopause; estradiol (E2)—predominant in nonpregnant females and most potent form; estriol (E3)—predominant in pregnancy; and estetrol (E4), produced solely in pregnancy.

Primarily estrogen production occurs in the ovary, but also can occur in adrenal and other sites like adipose tissue, skin fibroblasts, brain, bone, and placental syncytiotrophoblast through the enzyme aromatase which is a catalyst in the conversion of C19 steroids to estradiol.[25]

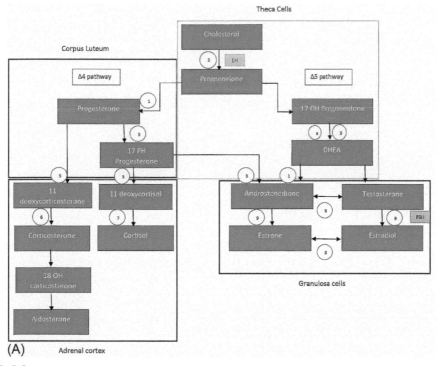

FIG. 2.8

(A) Ovarian steroidogenesis: (1) 3β-hydroxysteroid dehydrogenase; (2) CYP 11A; (3) CYP 17; (4) 17.20 lyase; (5) CYP 21; (6) CYP 11; (7) CYP 11 B1; (8) 17BHSB; (9) CYP 19. Role of the adrenal gland cortex has also been included.

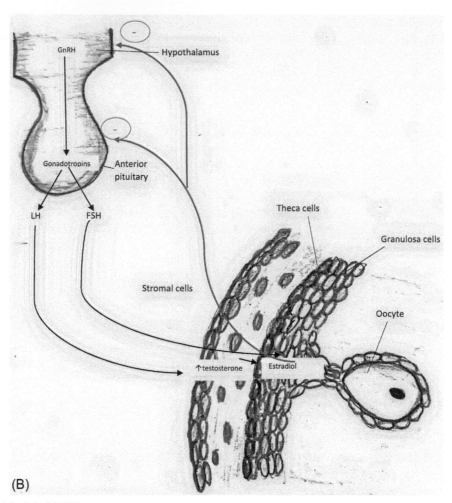

(B)

FIG. 2.8, CONT'D

(B) Hypothalamic–pituitary–ovarian axis, showing hormonal control of steroidogenesis. Pulsatile gonadotropin-releasing hormone (GnRH) release from hypothalamus stimulates luteinizing hormone (LH) and follicular-stimulating hormone (FSH) release from anterior pituitary. LH stimulates testosterone production from theca cells, which, in turn through aromatase, is converted to estradiol. Estradiol has negative feedback on anterior pituitary and hypothalamus.

Estradiol is produced by the granulosa cells in preovulatory follicles, from androstenedione produced by theca cells in the first half of the menstrual cycle, rate-limiting step being FSH-dependent aromatase regulation, and by corpus luteum in the latter half, under influence of FSH and LH. Cholesterol, the precursor for ovarian steroidogenesis, is derived from de novo synthesis in ovary, plasma lipoproteins, and lipid droplets containing cholesterol esters.

Estrogen works through its two distinct nuclear receptors: estrogen receptor alpha (ERα) found mainly in the uterus and pituitary gland, but also in liver, hypothalamus, bone, mammary gland, cervix, and vagina; estrogen receptor beta (ERβ), found primarily in ovarian granulosa cells, also in lung and prostate (in males).[26]

Functions of estrogen and progesterone are summarized in Table 2.3.

Table 2.3 Functions of estrogens and progesterone in various organs.

Organ	Function of estrogens	Function of progesterone
Hypothalamus	Regulation of GnRH production by feedback mechanism. Estradiol increases GnRH pulse frequency[27]	Progesterone reduces GnRH pulsatility and pulse frequency, leading to increased FSH in the late luteal phase - Increases hypothalamic temperature during luteal phase
Anterior pituitary	Regulation of FSH and LH production by negative feedback mechanisms - Stimulates LH surge preovulation	Regulation of FSH and LH production by negative feedback mechanisms
Uterus and cervix	- Thickening of endometrial tissues by rapid proliferation of stromal and epithelial cells - Increased responsiveness to progesterone receptors - Thinning of cervical mucus	- Endometrial cell differentiation and secretory activity induction after estrogen-priming of the uterus - Necessary for the implantation of fertilized ovum and pregnancy maintenance - Induces decidualization of endometrium - Prevents uterine contractions - Increases cervical mucus viscosity
Ovary	- Ovulation stimulation by increasing LH release	- Ovulation and luteinization[28]
Breast	Alongside GH and IGF-1, estrogen stimulates pubertal breast development and pregnancy-related breast maturation in preparation for lactation - Stimulates ductal production alongside fat and connective tissue depositions - Increases progesterone and prolactin receptors in breasts, thus indirectly promoting lobuloalveolar development[29]	Promotes lateral (lobuloalveolar) development - Inhibits lactation during pregnancy

Continued

Table 2.3 Functions of estrogens and progesterone in various organs—cont'd

Organ	Function of estrogens	Function of progesterone
Vagina	- Increased lubrication - Thickening of vaginal wall	
Musculoskeletal	- Growth spurt - Epiphyseal closure - Reduce bone resorption - Increase bone formation and mineralization	- Increased muscle mass
Brain	- Regulation of cognitive functions due to antiinflammatory effects[30] - Regulates DNA repair mechanisms in brain thus important for neuroprotection[31] - Mood and mental well-being regulation - Prevention of binge eating[32]	- Progesterone is a neurosteroid - Important for neuromodulation with a protective effect on damaged brain tissue - Regulate cognition, mood, and inflammation[33]
Libido	- Improved sex drive	- Decreased female sexual motivation
Metabolism and cardiovascular risk	High risk of impaired glucose tolerance, type 2 DM, and dyslipidemia in postmenopausal women with increased cardiovascular risk[34] - Increased hepatic protein production - Maintenance of skin and blood vessels	Reduce QT interval, increase NO levels, and influence cardiac repolarization, with reduced cardiac myocyte apoptosis[35]
Secondary sexual characteristics	Breast development, hip enlargement, female fat deposition during puberty	
Immunity	Antiinflammatory properties help mobilization of neutrophils[36]	During pregnancy, decreases maternal immune response to allow for pregnancy acceptance
Fluid and electrolyte balance	Increases sodium and water retention, increases SHBG and cortisol levels	Antimineralocorticoid effects stimulate natriuresis
Skin	Increased collagen, elasticity, and thickness, with improved hydration and surface lipids[37]	Increased collagen, elasticity, and thickness, with improved hydration and surface lipids

Progesterone

Progesterone is primarily produced by the corpus luteum, from pregnenolone, during the second half of the menstrual cycle. LDL-derived cholesterol is mainly utilized for progesterone production from granulosa lutein cells of corpus luteum and the rate-limiting step is access to cholesterol by the corpus luteal mitochondrial system.[38] Progesterone acts through classical nuclear receptors (PRα and PRβ) to induce transcription, and through nonclassical receptors (PQMR and PGMR1).

Progesterone acts as antiestrogen by reducing ERα expression, inducing 17βHSD2, thus increasing the conversion of estradiol to estrone, and increasing sulfation leading to inactivation of estradiol.[39]

The menstrual cycle

Defined as the serial changes in uterine lining from shedding, rebuilding, and preparation for implantation, the menstrual cycle begins at puberty and ends at menopause. Normal cycle length varies from 21 to 32 days, on average 28 days, and begins with the first day of menstrual bleeding.[7] The two phases of menstrual cycle include proliferative and secretory phases as briefed later (discussed in more detail in Chapter 3):

Proliferative/follicular phase: This starts from day 0 to 14 of menstrual cycle, beginning from the onset of menses and culminating in ovulation.

After menses, the proliferative phase begins with increasing levels of 17-beta-estradiol stimulated by the upregulation of FSH receptors in the follicles. Estradiol promotes endometrial growth by increasing stroma and glandular proliferation and increased penetration of the endometrial spiral arteries. In this phase, the cervical mucus thins and becomes watery to facilitate sperm penetration in preparation for fertilization. One of the primordial follicles is recruited and matures to the Graafian follicle, ready for ovulation (discussed earlier). Prior to ovulation, mature Graafian follicle produces high estradiol levels, which, when reach above 200 pg/mL, provide a positive feedback for increased FSH and LH release from anterior pituitary, termed as the LH surge. This stimulates the release of the mature ovum by ovulation, followed by a drop in estradiol levels. The high estradiol also stimulates uterine tube contractions and uptake of the released ovum.[7]

Luteal/secretory phase: Occurring from day 14 to 28, this phase is predominantly mediated by progesterone produced from the corpus luteum postovulation and involves the preparation of the endometrium for implantation of a fertilized ovum. This phase involves increased secretion of glycogen-rich fluid from endometrial glands, necessary for energy provision to the developing zygote if implantation occurs. Progesterone also increases vascular supply to the stratum functionalis layer. The cervical mucus is decreased and thickens since sperm permeability is not a high consideration at this stage. If fertilization does not occur, the levels of estradiol and progesterone drop significantly and menses occur.

Menses

With low levels of estradiol and progesterone, the endometrium lining, stratum functionalis, loses its blood supply due to increased prostaglandin release and is shed off as menses. The low levels of steroid hormones stimulate the release of FSH and LH from the anterior pituitary and the cycle repeats.

Menopause

Menopause is the cessation of the menstrual cycle due to the loss of ovarian follicles and hence steroidogenic capacity, ranging from 50 to 52 years of age, and considered complete after 1 year of amenorrhea.[7] While approaching menopause, inhibin production reduces and its levels decline from the ovary, thus increasing FSH production by negative feedback, which in turn increases estrogen production from secondary follicles. Eventually, these undergo atresia until no more follicles exist, thus the drop in estrogen levels and symptoms of menopause setting in. Of note is that LH levels remain relatively steady and thus testosterone and androstenedione production continue in the ovary, with DHEA/DHEAS production ongoing in the adrenal glands. Androstenedione is converted to estrone by aromatase enzyme and estrone is converted peripherally to estradiol.

Perimenopause is the transition to menopause in which hormonal and psychosomatic changes occur and is marked by irregular menstrual bleeding, mostly with increased cycle lengths.

Symptoms of menopause, occurring in varying severity within different females, include hot flashes, sweats, urogenital atrophy presented as dyspareunia and urinary difficulties, osteoporosis, and increased CVD risk.

Female sexual response

Female sexual response is divided into four stages: excitement, arousal, plateau/orgasm, and resolution.[40] The biophysiological model of female sexual response includes an interplay of biological factors (e.g., physical health, neurobiology, and endocrine function), psychological health (e.g., performance anxiety, and depression), interpersonal factors (e.g., relationship quality, life stressors, abstinence intervals, and finances), and sociocultural factors (e.g., upbringing, cultural norms, and expectations) that influence desire.[41] Factors such as images, scent, music, fantasy trigger excitement, which is mediated by neuroendocrine systems in the brain.[42]

In the **arousal phase**, there is increased estrogen responsiveness with increased vaginal blood flow and lubrication. The labia, vagina, and clitoris get engorged with blood (genital vasocongestion), vulval swelling exposes introitus, vagina lengthens and dilates with tightening of the outer part, clitoris' length and diameter increase, which is then followed by the plateau/orgasm phase, comprising vaginal, uterine, and levator ani muscle rhythmic contractions, causing a sense of release for the woman.[43] This is followed by resolution stage, where blood flow decreases to sexual organs and muscles relax, giving a relaxed, euphoric, and satisfied feeling.[44]

In women, erection does not occur due to the thinner tunica which cannot trap venous blood unlike in males.[45] Central excitatory factors include estrogen, testosterone, melanocortin, oxytocin, dopamine, and norepinephrine, whereas inhibitory factors are serotonin, prolactin, and opioids.[45]

Interplay of female endocrine and reproductive systems

As in males, the hypothalamus in females produces GnRH from the arcuate nucleus in a pulsatile manner beginning from its maturity at puberty and regulates the secretion of anterior pituitary hormones FSH and LH, by its release through the hypothalamo-pituitary portal system (Fig. 2.8B).

GnRH release is affected by various factors including ovarian steroids, dopamine, serotonin, and opioids. Estradiol and norepinephrine stimulate GnRH release, whereas progesterone, dopamine, beta-endorphins, and other opioids suppress its release.[27] Kisspeptins also stimulate GnRH release and are essential for sexual development and function.[46]

GnRH stimulates the release of FSH and LH from anterior pituitary gonadotroph cells. The release of FSH and LH is also modulated by estradiol; progesterone and the peptide inhibin of ovarian origin; activin and follistatin of pituitary origin. Estradiol and inhibin have suppressive effects on FSH, whereas activin stimulates its release. Follistatin inhibits activin action, thus inhibits FSH production, and releases indirectly.

LH primarily stimulates theca cell androstenedione production, whereas FSH controls follicular growth and granulosa cell production of estradiol and inhibin B. After ovulation (mediated by the LH surge), LH stimulates estrogen, progesterone, and inhibin A production by corpus luteum.[47]

Conclusions

The male and female reproductive systems are a complex interplay of structural and neuroendocrine processes that are initiated in utero as a part of normal embryonic development, proceed to mature with increasing age, marking the onset and progress of puberty, which is indicative of both internal and external sexual maturity. The final goal is to ensure the maintenance of normal secondary sex characteristics and ensure procreation. Disturbances in the physiology of the reproductive systems thus form a significant cause of male- and female-related subfertility/infertility.

References

1. Turek PJ. Male reproductive physiology. In: Wein AJ, Kavoussi LR, Novick AC, Partin AW, Peters AP, eds. *Campbell-Walsh Urology*. 22. 11th ed. Philadelphia: Elsevier-Saunders; 2015:516–537.e5.
2. O'Donnell L, Stanton P, de Kretser DM. Endocrinology of the male reproductive system and spermatogenesis. In: *Endotext [Internet]*. MDText.com, Inc; 2017. https://www.ncbi.nlm.nih.gov/books/NBK279031/. Accessed: 19.02.2020.
3. Robert CD, Tom FL. Physiology of penile erection and pathophysiology of erectile dysfunction. *Urol Clin North Am*. 2005;32(4):379–403.

4. Mulhall JP, Incrocci L, Goldstein I, Rosen R, eds. *Cancer and Sexual Health.* Springer Science & Business Media; 2011. https://books.google.com.pk/books?hl=en&lr=&id=GpIadil3YsQC&oi=fnd&pg=PR3&dq=Mulhall+JP,+2011.+Cancer+and+sexual+health.+Springer+Science+%26+Business+Media.&ots=TJgLoEdvZc&sig=ybIKJHiLwLgF5zGJMza7d48mTxg&redir_esc=y#v=onepage&q=Mulhall%20JP%2C%202011.%20Cancer%20and%20sexual%20health.%20Springer%20Science%20%26%20Business%20Media.&f=false. Accessed: 19.02.2020.

5. Comarr AE. Sexual function among patients with spinal cord injury. *Urol Int.* 1970;25(2):134–168. https://doi.org/10.1159/000279669.

6. DeGroat WC, Booth AM. Physiology of male sexual function. *Ann Intern Med.* 1980;92(2 pt. 2):329–331. https://doi.org/10.7326/0003-4819-92-2-329.

7. Bulun SE. Physiology and pathology of the female reproductive axis. In: Kronenberg HM, Melmed S, Polonsky KS, Larsen PR, eds. *Williams Textbook of Endocrinology.* 14th ed. Philadelphia: Elsevier Health Sciences; 2020:574–641.e10. https://www.clinicalkey.com/#!/content/book/3-s2.0-B9780323555968000176?scrollTo=%23top. Accessed: 20.02.2020.

8. Handelsman DJ. Androgen physiology, pharmacology and abuse. In: Feingold KR, Anawalt B, Boyce A, et al., eds. *Endotext [Internet].* South Dartmouth, MA: MDText.com, Inc; 2000. Available from https://www.ncbi.nlm.nih.gov/books/NBK279000/. Accessed: 05.06.2020.

9. Wu FC, Butler GE, Kelnar CJ, Sellar RE. Patterns of pulsatile luteinizing hormone secretion before and during the onset of puberty in boys: a study using an immunoradiometric assay. *J Clin Endocrinol Metab.* 1990;70(3):629–637. https://doi.org/10.1210/jcem-70-3-629.

10. Sanfilippo JS, Jamieson MA. Physiology of puberty. *Gynecol Obstet.* 2008. http://bezak.umms.med.umich.edu/CIRHT/Content/Gynaecology%20and%20Obstetrics%20-%20Open%20Textbooks/BookCh-Physiology%20of%20Puberty-GLOWM-CustomLicense.pdf. Accessed: 19.02.2020.

11. Alotaibi MF. Physiology of puberty in boys and girls and pathological disorders affecting its onset. *J Adolesc.* 2019;71:63–71. https://doi.org/10.1016/j.adolescence.2018.12.007.

12. Cheng G, Coolen LM, Padmanabhan V, Goodman RL, Lehman MN. The kisspeptin/neurokinin B/dynorphin (KNDy) cell population of the arcuate nucleus: sex differences and effects of prenatal testosterone in sheep. *Endocrinology.* 2010;151(1):301–311. https://doi.org/10.1210/en.2009-0541.

13. Marshall WA, Tanner JM. Variations in the pattern of pubertal changes in boys. *Arch Dis Child.* 1970;45(239):13–23. https://doi.org/10.1136/adc.45.239.13.

14. Rojas J, Chávez-Castillo M, Olivar LC, et al. Physiologic course of female reproductive function: a molecular look into the prologue of life. *J Pregnancy.* 2015;2015. https://doi.org/10.1155/2015/715735.

15. Nguyen J, Duong H. Anatomy, abdomen and pelvis, female external genitalia. In: *StatPearls.* Treasure Island, FL: StatPearls Publishing; 2020. https://www.ncbi.nlm.nih.gov/books/NBK547703/. Accessed: 12.01.2020.

16. Edson MA, Nagaraja AK, Matzuk MM. The mammalian ovary from genesis to revelation. *Endocr Rev.* 2009;30(6):624–712. https://doi.org/10.1210/er.2009-0012.

17. Elmlinger MW, Kühnel W, Wormstall H, Döller PC. Reference intervals for testosterone, androstenedione and SHBG levels in healthy females and males from birth until old age. *Clin Lab.* 2005;51(11–12):625–632. https://pubmed.ncbi.nlm.nih.gov/16329620/. Accessed: 05.06.2020.

18. Oktem O, Oktay K. The ovary: anatomy and function throughout human life. *Ann NY Acad Sci.* 2008;1127:1–9. https://doi.org/10.1196/annals.1434.009.

19. Himelstein-Braw R, Byskov AG, Peters H, Faber M. Follicular atresia in the infant human ovary. *J Reprod Fertil.* 1976;46(1):55–59. https://doi.org/10.1530/jrf.0.0460055.

20. Ohara A, Mori T, Taii S, Ban C, Narimoto K. Functional differentiation in steroidogenesis of two types of luteal cells isolated from mature human corpora lutea of menstrual cycle. *J Clin Endocrinol Metab.* 1987;65(6):1192–1200. https://doi.org/10.1210/jcem-65-6-1192.

21. Duncan WC, McNeilly AS, Fraser HM, Illingworth PJ. Luteinizing hormone receptor in the human corpus luteum: lack of down-regulation during maternal recognition of pregnancy. *Hum Reprod.* 1996;11(10):2291–2297. https://doi.org/10.1093/oxfordjournals.humrep.a019091.

22. Tilly JL, Kowalski KI, Johnson AL, Hsueh AJ. Involvement of apoptosis in ovarian follicular atresia and postovulatory regression. *Endocrinology.* 1991;129(5):2799–2801. https://doi.org/10.1210/endo-129-5-2799.

23. Magnusson C, Billig H, Eneroth P, Roos P, Hillensjö T. Comparison between the progestin secretion responsiveness to gonadotrophins of rat cumulus and mural granulosa cells in vitro. *Acta Endocrinol.* 1982;101(4):611–616. https://doi.org/10.1530/acta.0.1010611.

24. Erickson GF, Magoffin DA, Dyer CA, Hofeditz C. The ovarian androgen producing cells: a review of structure/function relationships. *Endocr Rev.* 1985;6(3):371–399. https://doi.org/10.1210/edrv-6-3-371.

25. Nelson LR, Bulun SE. Estrogen production and action. *J Am Acad Dermatol.* 2001;45(3 suppl):S116–S124. https://doi.org/10.1067/mjd.2001.117432.

26. Hamilton KJ, Hewitt SC, Arao Y, Korach KS. Estrogen hormone biology. In: *Current Topics in Developmental Biology.* vol. 125. Academic Press; 2017:109–146. https://www.sciencedirect.com/science/article/abs/pii/S0070215316302046. Accessed: 20.02.2020.

27. Haisenleder DJ, Dalkin AC, Ortolano GA, Marshall JC, Shupnik MA. A pulsatile gonadotropin-releasing hormone stimulus is required to increase transcription of the gonadotropin subunit genes: evidence for differential regulation of transcription by pulse frequency in vivo. *Endocrinology.* 1991;128(1):509–517. https://doi.org/10.1210/endo-128-1-509.

28. Suzuki T, Sasano H, Kimura N, et al. Immunohistochemical distribution of progesterone, androgen and oestrogen receptors in the human ovary during the menstrual cycle: relationship to expression of steroidogenic enzymes. *Hum Reprod.* 1994;9(9):1589–1595. https://doi.org/10.1093/oxfordjournals.humrep.a138757.

29. Coad J, Dunstall M. *Anatomy and Physiology for Midwives e-Book.* Elsevier Health Sciences; 2011. https://books.google.com.pk/books?hl=en&lr=&id=95kqFLm3UfMC&oi=fnd&pg=PP1&dq=Coad+J,+Dunstall+M.+Anatomy+and+physiology+for+midwives+e-book.+Elsevier+Health+Sciences%3B+2011+Jun+10.&ots=-FL33XTukt&sig=TngwxpV02-5g10BFBpacySHYFkk&redir_esc=y#v=onepage&q&f=false. Accessed: 20.02.2020.

30. Au A, Feher A, McPhee L, Jessa A, Oh S, Einstein G. Estrogens, inflammation and cognition. *Front Neuroendocrinol.* 2016;40:87–100. https://doi.org/10.1016/j.yfrne.2016.01.002.

31. Zárate S, Stevnsner T, Gredilla R. Role of estrogen and other sex hormones in brain aging. Neuroprotection and DNA repair. *Front Aging Neurosci.* 2017;9:430. https://doi.org/10.3389/fnagi.2017.00430.

32. Klump KL, Racine SE, Hildebrandt B, et al. Ovarian hormone influences on dysregulated eating: a comparison of associations in women with versus without binge episodes. *Clin Psychol Sci.* 2014;2(4):545–559. https://doi.org/10.1177/2167702614521794.

33. Brinton RD, Thompson RF, Foy MR, et al. Progesterone receptors: form and function in brain. *Front Neuroendocrinol.* 2008;29(2):313–339. https://doi.org/10.1016/j.yfrne.2008.02.001.

34. Munoz J, Derstine A, Gower BA. Fat distribution and insulin sensitivity in postmeno-pausal women: influence of hormone replacement. *Obes Res.* 2002;10(6):424–431. https://doi.org/10.1038/oby.2002.59.

35. Исаева АС. Non-reproductive system effects of progesterone and its non-selective antagonists mifepristone. *Reprod Endocrinol.* 2017;(33):8–16. https://doi.org/10.18370/2309-4117.2017.33.8-16.

36. Nadkarni S, Cooper D, Brancaleone V, Bena S, Perretti M. Activation of the annexin A1 pathway underlies the protective effects exerted by estrogen in polymorphonuclear leuko-cytes. *Arterioscler Thromb Vasc Biol.* 2011;31(11):2749–2759. https://doi.org/10.1161/ATVBAHA.111.235176.

37. Holzer G, Riegler E, Hönigsmann H, Farokhnia S, Schmidt JB. Effects and side-effects of 2% progesterone cream on the skin of peri- and postmenopausal women: results from a double-blind, vehicle-controlled, randomized study [published correction appears in Br J Dermatol. 2005 Nov;153(5):1092. Schmidt, B [corrected to Schmidt, JB]]. *Br J Dermatol.* 2005;153(3):626–634. https://doi.org/10.1111/j.1365-2133.2005.06685.x.

38. Carr BR, MacDonald PC, Simpson ER. The role of lipoproteins in the regulation of progesterone secretion by the human corpus luteum. *Fertil Steril.* 1982;38(3):303–311. https://doi.org/10.1016/s0015-0282(16)46511-8.

39. Yang S, Fang Z, Gurates B, et al. Stromal PRs mediate induction of 17beta-hydroxysteroid dehydrogenase type 2 expression in human endometrial epithelium: a paracrine mech-anism for inactivation of E2. *Mol Endocrinol.* 2001;15(12):2093–2105. https://doi.org/10.1210/mend.15.12.0742.

40. Rao TS, Nagaraj AK. Female sexuality. *Indian J Psychiatry.* 2015;57(suppl. 2):S296–S302. https://doi.org/10.4103/0019-5545.161496.

41. Levine SB. The nature of sexual desire: a clinician's perspective. *Arch Sex Behav.* 2003;32(3):279–285. https://doi.org/10.1023/a:1023421819465.

42. Arcos B. Female sexual function and response. *J Am Osteopath Assoc.* 2004;104(1 suppl. 1):S16–S20. https://jaoa.org/article.aspx?articleid=2092848. Accessed: 06.06.2020.

43. Kim JH. Urogynecology and reconstructive pelvic surgery. 4th ed. *Int Neurourol J.* 2015;19(1):51. https://doi.org/10.5213/inj.2015.19.1.51.

44. Basson R. Women's sexual dysfunction: revised and expanded definitions. *CMAJ.* 2005;172(10):1327–1333. https://doi.org/10.1503/cmaj.1020174.

45. Perelman MA. The sexual tipping point: a mind/body model for sexual medicine. *J Sex Med.* 2009;6(3):629–632. https://doi.org/10.1111/j.1743-6109.2008.01177.x.

46. Seminara SB, Messager S, Chatzidaki EE, et al. The GPR54 gene as a regulator of pu-berty. *N Engl J Med.* 2003;349(17):1614–1627. https://doi.org/10.1056/NEJMoa035322.

47. Hall JE. *Guyton & Hall Physiology Review e-Book.* 3rd ed. Elsevier Health Sciences; 2015. https://www.elsevier.com/books/guyton-and-hall-physiology-review/hall/978-1-4557-7007-6.

Reproductive cycle

3

Rabiya Ali[a,b] and Rehana Rehman[c]

[a]Department of Physiology, Karachi Institute of Medical Sciences (KIMS), CMH, Karachi, Pakistan, [b]Department of Physiology, University of Karachi, Karachi, Pakistan, [c]Department of Biological & Biomedical Sciences, Aga Khan University, Karachi, Pakistan

Chapter outline

Introduction

Every healthy human female experiences reproductive cycles that organize their reproductive system for pregnancy. The reproductive cycles are under the dynamic influence of integrated action of hormones from hypothalamus, anterior pituitary, and gonadal ovarian steroids. Ovarian cycle is directly regulated and synchronized by the anterior pituitary follicle-stimulating hormone (FSH) and luteinizing hormone (LH). Uterine cycle is controlled by a direct reaction to ovarian steroid hormones

Subfertility. https://doi.org/10.1016/B978-0-323-75945-8.00003-7

(estrogen and progesterone).[1] The definitive rheostat of the pituitary gonadotropins (FSH and LH) is situated centrally in the hypothalamus, which is highly responsive to plasma concentration of ovarian steroid hormones. The gonadotropin synthesis and secretion from anterior pituitary are augmented and regulated by the release of gonadotropin-releasing hormone (GnRH) from hypothalamus into hypothalamic–hypophyseal–portal circulation.[1]

Puberty in females
An overview of menarche

In girls, puberty is considered as the development of the genital organs, secondary sexual characteristics, and the appearance of menarche.[2] Thus, the main physiological mechanisms that determine puberty in girls include ovarian growth and maturation with increased synthesis and secretion of sex steroid hormones with folliculogenesis and ovulation. These changes are responsible for the occurrence of menarche in girls.[3] Menarche is the memorable beginning of a woman's reproductive life. It is commonly accepted that the cyclical hormonal variabilities that control the reproductive cycle have an essential natural impact on a woman's physical and mental health.[4] This cycle duration is from 25 to 35 days, usually of 28 and 26 days of length in women's reproductive life.[5] The usual age group at menarche is 9–14 years and the mean is 12–13 years. Body mass index and lifestyle may influence the age at menarche.[3,6] Menarche is associated with an anovulatory cycle and ideally appears 2–2.5 years after the initial stages of mammary gland development. In the 1st year postmenarche, the menstrual cycles are typically irregular and anovulatory ranges from 21 to 45 days.[7] Menstrual cycles can remain continuously irregular until the 3–5th year postmenarche.[7] The predominance of primordial and preantral follicles occurs before puberty; tiny follicles can grow through this period of development. These small follicles are gonadotropin-independent. The volume of ovary increases by the commencement of adolescence, attains increase in bulk or size rapidly after menarche especially between 13 and 16 years, and remains constant or decreased marginally subsequently. Polycystic ovarian morphological changes are noticed in healthy young girls; this morphology is not associated with reduced ovulatory rate, hyperandrogenism, or metabolic disorders.[8] In the initial phase of postmenarche, ovarian morphological changes on transabdominal ultrasound scan show multicystic ovaries and significantly raised ovarian volume that differs from ovarian morphological features observed in elder women.[9]

The menstrual cycle

In the normal ovulatory menstrual cycle, four hormones FSH, LH, estrogen, and progesterone, with the central pulsatile release of GnRH, regulate the normal reproductive activities in women like continuous cycles of follicular growth and development, ovulation, and endometrial preparation for the implantation of the blastocyst (Fig. 3.1). Active high secretion of FSH through the luteal–follicular

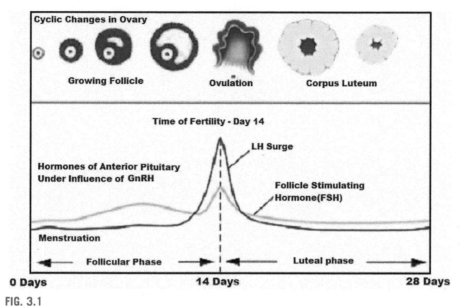

FIG. 3.1

Reproductive cycle.

From Koyama A, Hagopian L, Linden J. Emerging options for emergency contraception. Clin Med Insights Reprod Health. 2013:7;CMRH-S8145.

switch leads to the staffing of a troop of follicles and the appearance and progression of a dominant follicle called mature Graafian follicle. From the ovary, estradiol and inhibin release are the main inhibitors of ongoing excitatory release of FSH, while high estradiol with other prospective elements is significant for the LH surge, centrally regulated at anterior pituitary in women.[10] Corpus luteum releases progesterone and estradiol to prepare the uterine endometrium for implantation, and its decease permits FSH to become high with the start of a next cycle.[10]

The phases of menstrual cycle with endocrine control
Follicular phase

Early follicular period is best described as "an early rise in FSH with mobilization of fresh follicular squad toward the growing bank of follicles with high secretions of inhibin B and an initial rise in estradiol levels." The initial part of the follicular phase of the well-maintained cycle is significantly associated with obvious declining of GnRH pulsatile release during sleep.[11] Sleep may cause a fall in pulsatile GnRH release from hypothalamus (Fig. 3.2) and may assist the role of maintaining FSH synthesis during this sensitive phase of follicular trooping.[12]

The middle part of follicular phase is mainly characterized by the dominant follicle appearance and lower secretion of FSH in response to inhibin B and high estradiol concentration with a later high level of inhibin A. High estradiol causes

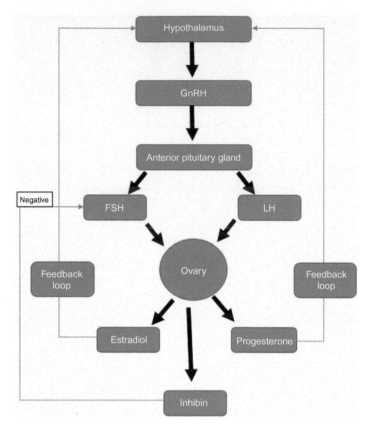

FIG. 3.2

Hypothalamic–pituitary–ovarian axis.

endometrial growth and development. In the mid-follicular period, GnRH pulsa-tile release becomes high and interpulse break minimizes to almost 1 h. LH pulse amplitude is significantly reduced, demonstrating the downregulation (negative feedback) of estradiol release from growing follicles in response to the GnRH pulse amplitude and due to the straight anterior pituitary suppression of gonadotrope re-lease.[12] The latter part of the follicular period is best described by rapid and in-creased secretion of estradiol and inhibin A in association with inhibin B and FSH decreased concentrations. The cyclical discharge of GnRH that started at the mid-follicular period is sustained to the latter part of the follicular phase. However, LH secretion increases as a result of the excitatory signaling from high estradiol and possibly inhibin A on gonadotropes, with increased responsiveness to GnRH. This significant increase in estradiol levels is responsible for active endometrial growth and proliferation.[13]

Mid-cycle surge

Due to exponential high estradiol and possibly inhibin A secretion in the late follicular phase, LH concentration increases 10-fold in 48–72 h, while FSH concentration raises 4-fold. The LH surge in the middle cycle is mainly needed for final oocyte maturation and start of follicular rupture, commonly ensuing almost 36 h post-LH surge. LH surge is widely accepted as a crucial factor for normal regular reproductive cycles. The levels for estrogen secretion are sensitive to positive feedback. Recommendations of synthetic estradiol to healthy ladies at the time of initial follicular phase[13] or to postmenopausal women[14] prompt rise in basal and GnRH induced LH release, which is more reliant on the dosage and extent of estrogen secretion. The high estradiol always favors the LH surge.[13]

Luteal phase

After ovulation, the development of corpus luteum results in the discharge of progesterone, estradiol, and inhibin A and generates suppressive effects on gonadotropins (FSH, LH) release. Reduced pulsatile GnRH secretion starts at the end of the mid-cycle surge and lasts throughout the luteal phase; this effect occurs due to progesterone. In the luteal phase, LH pulse rates are highly expressive as compared to the follicular phase due to reduced pulsatile GnRH secretion induced by progesterone and the inverse association among LH sensitivity to GnRH and GnRH pulse frequency[15] and also due to the direct effect of progesterone on the anterior pituitary to enhance LH sensitivity to GnRH.[16] The corpus luteum has a limited life, and during the nonexistence of gestation, reduced blood concentration of progesterone and estradiol leads to endometrial shedding.[17]

Luteal–follicular transition

The weakening of corpus luteum and reduced secretion of ovarian steroid hormones and inhibin A facilitates increased FSH secretion that starts before menstruation and participates in the accumulation of fresh troop of follicles in the emerging bank. Maintenance of the mid-luteal-period concentration of estradiol controls rise in FSH.[17] While proof for the effect of estradiol in the negative feedback control of FSH secretion in women is well established , the role of inhibins A and B relative to estradiol and relative to each other remains disputed. Control of the FSH rise across the luteal–follicular transition is regulated in part by release of negative feedback associated with deteriorating levels of estradiol from the decease of the corpus luteum. Therefore, scientists investigated the effects of tamoxifen to suppress the estrogen receptor in normal cycles explored that inhibin A participates in preventing the FSH release through normal luteal phase.[17] LH pulse frequency raises just prior to the start of menstrual discharge. LH pulse frequency is negatively associated with progesterone levels, and administering the mid-luteal-period quantities of progesterone in combination with estradiol controls normal luteal–follicular rise in GnRH pulse frequency in healthy women.[18]

Histological changes during menstrual cycle
Early proliferative phase

In the early proliferative period, the endometrial width is normally <2 mm. In lower basal zones, the multiplication of cells occur and epithelial layers enduring in the basal uterine divisions lead to renovation and luminal epithelium repair through day 5 of the normal cycle. During this, mitosis is apparent in the glandular and stromal epithelial lining. This frequent practice of wound healing generally avoided the scarring.[19] Endometrial stem cells are highly proficient in producing precursors of stromal and epithelial origins. Adult progenitor cells have the capacity to remarkably contribute to the regenerative process.[19,20] In the early proliferative phase, the endometrial glands are narrow and straight, with the lining of low columnar cells. The ultrastructure showed epithelial cell cytoplasm with several ribosomes; however, endoplasmic reticulum with Golgi apparatus is not well developed in these cells.[21]

Late proliferative phase

As an outcome of endometrial glandular hyperplasia and rise in stromal extracellular matrix, the thickness of endometrium improves in the late proliferative phase. The glands are extensively parted proximate to the surface of the endometrium and more congested and convoluted deeply into the endometrium. The glandular epithelial cells become tall and pseudostratified near ovulation. The impact of steroid hormones on endometrium growth, development, and secretion is mainly reliant on basalis and functionalis zones, and endometrial proliferation is confined to the functionalis layer.[21]

Early secretory phase

Ovulation indicates the commencement of secretory period of endometrial cycle, while it is distinguished, the endometrial luminal cells and glandular cells also demonstrate secretory action after the proliferative period. Mitotic events in epithelial and stromal cells are limited to initial 3 days postovulation and are hardly witnessed in the subsequent part of the cycle. Ultrastructural level of endometrial epithelia discloses plentiful endoplasmic reticulum, un-remarkably big-sized mitochondria with noticeable and dominant cristae. A network of collagen type 1 and collagen type 3 is recognized in stroma through early secretory period. Edematous changes in stroma contribute to the endometrial thickening during this time.

Mid-secretory phase

The distinguishing point of the mid-secretory period is the expansion of spiral arteries. These blood vessels become largely spiraled. The glands are tortuous with secretory function, reaches at a highest level 6 days postovulation, demonstrated through the absence of vacuoles from the epithelial cell cytoplasm, the nucleolar channel system, visible briefly in nucleoli of 10% of the secretory phase epithelial cells within 16–24 days.[22] The nuclear channel system comprises of amorphous matrix, dense granules, and a series of tubular channels. The nuclear channel system is the inward folding of the inner nuclear membrane, for the transport of mRNA to the cytoplasm.[23] The nucleolar channel system is an ultrastructure assurance of the secretory phase during implantation. The expansion of stromal cells around the vessel attains an eosinophilic cytoplasm with pericellular extracellular matrix in the mid-to-late secretory period. These modifications are called predecidualization to differentiate them from additional stromal alteration that arises in a fertile cycle, emphasizing the demarcation among the subepithelial compact and spongy zone.[24]

Decidual stromal cells contribute primarily in maternal–fetal interfaces and their precursors confine to the endometrial and decidual perivascular region where these precursors share the alpha-smooth muscle actin expression and contraction under the cytokine influence.[25] Ultrastructurally, the predecidual stromal cells show well established Golgi apparatus and endoplasmic reticulum. The laminin, fibronectin, heparan sulfate, and type IV collagen are parts of nearby matrix.[26,27] Stromal cells of the mid-secretory and late secretory phases express the protein stock that stimulates hemostasis by a tissue factor, a membrane-bound protein that starts blood coagulation once it comes in contact with ruptured blood vessel, blood, and plasminogen activator inhibitor type 1, which prevent fibrinolysis.[28]

Premenstrual and menstrual phase

Principal histologic characteristics of premenstrual duration are the extinction of stromal reticular nexus, assemble, or catalyzed by matrix metalloproteinase (MMPs) infiltration of stromal layer by polymorphonuclear and mononuclear leukocytes. The endometrial glands become fatigued and tired due to massive secretion, and epithelial cells show nuclei at the lowest regions. The nuclei of granular lymphocytes, undergo pyknosis and karyorrhexis indicating apoptosis, suggested as few initial events portend menses. These modifications occur before the degradation of the extracellular matrix and leukocytic penetration.[28] In the glandular epithelium, the nucleolar channel system, oversized mitochondria, and features of the early and mid-secretory periods are disappeared. The uterine endometrial lining reduces and paves the way for endometrial shedding in menstruation, partially due to the reduced secretory process and breakdown of the extracellular matrix.[29]

Menstruation

This phase mainly ensues by progesterone decline, sign of failure to attain conception, and necessity to remove the specialized uterine endometrial layer developed during decidualization.[29] The uniqueness of the phase is determined by progesterone and estrogen decline with corpus luteum deterioration. In infertile cycles, the menses appear nearly and exclusively in humans and some old primates. The molecular mechanisms activated as a result of progesterone decline involve the excitation of the nuclear factor kappa-light-chain-enhancer of activated B cell (NF-κβ) transcriptional pathway, a principal target of cytokines and subsequent genetic expression like endometrial bleeding-associated factor (EBAF), an anti-TGF-β cytokine that restricts the mechanism of action of other constitute of TGF-β family that endorses the endometrial rectitude. The coordinated blockage of the events of TGF-β seems to commence major succeeding measures of menses, comprising expansion of MMPs.[30]

Menstrual disturbances associated with the pathological conditions

Disturbance in the menstrual cycle may influence the reproductive life of young girls as well as adult women. The developing high prevalence of dysmenorrhea (painful menses), irregularity in monthly cycles, prolonged heavy menstrual bleeding in young girls and adult women is associated with a significant amount of physical and mental stress. Dysmenorrhea restricts their routine physical activities and affects the quality of life.[31] Dysmenorrhea may be of primary/unknown origin or secondary when there is an identified underlying cause.[32] Endometriosis is considered the commonest reason for painful menstruation.[33] Regular exercise, early childbirth, and proper management can help to control dysmenorrhea and chances of related complications in these girls.[33]

The lengthy interval between the cycles and heavy menstruation are alarming features when associated with anovulation, hirsutism, and acne.[34] Cushing syndrome, thyroid disorders, adrenal abnormalities, ovarian tumors, and premature decline in ovaries are the common pathological conditions associated with oligomenorrhea,[35] which refer to the occurrence of menses at intervals of more than 35 days due to a prolonged follicular phase. Oligomenorrhea needs logical evaluation and treatment, regardless of age.[6] Oligomenorrhea in young girls is significantly associated with hyperandrogenism and insulin resistance, the hallmark of the polycystic ovarian syndrome (PCOS).[36] Amenorrhea (primary and secondary) is also a common problem among girls and adult women. Primary amenorrhea means menarche fails to arise and secondary amenorrhea means the termination of menses after the commencement. These problems in young females are mainly because of the instabilities of the hypothalamic–pituitary–ovarian axis (H–P–O axis).[37] The variation in prognosis from females with secondary amenorrhea, compared with females having a history of oligomenorrhea indicates diverse mechanisms responsible for the malfunctioning of menstrual cycle. Hypothalamic suppression of the ovarian axis leads to secondary amenorrhea, while hyperandrogenism and PCOS are commonly observed in girls with oligomenorrhea.[8] The majority of cases (61%) of PCOS present with oligomenorrhea at their first visit. Hence, it is suggested that menstrual irregularities with the reduced menstrual flow in young girls are an initial alarming signal for PCOS.[36,38]

Menorrhagia refers to the heavy bleeding of more than 80 mL with passage of clots, occurring at normal intervals (from 21 to 35 days) and the duration of flow for more than a week.[35] Such a problem is mostly seen in young girls and adult women with frequent bruising due to inherited coagulopathy; in these situations, consultation with a hematologist should be considered an essential step in the absence of suitable screening tests for underlying disorders.[35] Polymenorrhea refers to the luteal-phase defects, which results in shortened cycles (<21 days).[35] Menorrhagia and polymenorrhea are the characteristic features of dysfunctional uterine bleeding (DUB), which is not associated with gestation or any systemic disorder and needs emergency care.[35,39] The actual underlying mechanism is unidentified, but it may be due to abnormal ovarian steroid hormone levels, disruption of the H–P–O axis that results in menstrual irregularities after menarche, or particularly during perimenopausal years when deteriorating secretions of estrogen remain unsuccessful to achieve LH surge and ovulation.[39] Irregular bleeding and spotting between periods are also associated with DUB.[39]

References

1. Maggi R, Cariboni AM, Marelli MM, et al. GnRH and GnRH receptors in the pathophysiology of the human female reproductive system. *Hum Reprod Update.* 2016;22(3):358–381.
2. Webster N, Gove PB. *Webster's Third New International Dictionary.* Bell; 1961.
3. Palmert MR, Dunkel L. Delayed puberty. *N Engl J Med.* 2012;366:443–453.
4. Farage MA, Neill S, MacLean AB. Physiological changes associated with the menstrual cycle: a review. *Obstet Gynecol Surv.* 2009;64(1):58–72.
5. Baker FC, Driver HS. Circadian rhythms, sleep, and the menstrual cycle. *Sleep Med.* 2007;8(6):613–622.
6. Rigon F, De Sanctis V, Bernasconi S, et al. Menstrual pattern and menstrual disorders among adolescents: an update of the Italian data. *Ital J Pediatr.* 2012;38(1):38.
7. Legro RS, Lin HM, Demers LM, Lloyd T. Rapid maturation of the reproductive axis during perimenarche independent of body composition. *J Clin Endocrinol Metabol.* 2000;85(3):1021–1025.
8. Codner E, Villarroel C, Eyzaguirre FC, et al. Polycystic ovarian morphology in postmenarchal adolescents. *Fertil Steril.* 2011;95(2):702–706.e702.
9. Hickey M, Doherty D, Atkinson H, et al. Clinical, ultrasound and biochemical features of polycystic ovary syndrome in adolescents: implications for diagnosis. *Hum Reprod.* 2011;26(6):1469–1477.
10. Treloar AE, Boynton RE, Behn BG, Brown BW. Variation of the human menstrual cycle through reproductive life. *Int J Fertil.* 1967;12(1 Pt 2):77–126.

11. Hall JE, Sullivan JP, Richardson GS. Brief wake episodes modulate sleep-inhibited luteinizing hormone secretion in the early follicular phase. *J Clin Endocrinol Metabol.* 2005;90(4):2050–2055.

12. Hall JE, Taylor A, Hayes F, Crowley W. Insights into hypothalamic-pituitary dysfunction in polycystic ovary syndrome. *J Endocrinol Invest.* 1998;21(9):602–611.

13. Taylor A, Whitney H, Hall JE, Martin K, Crowley Jr WF. Midcycle levels of sex steroids are sufficient to recreate the follicle-stimulating hormone but not the luteinizing hormone midcycle surge: evidence for the contribution of other ovarian factors to the surge in normal women. *J Clin Endocrinol Metabol.* 1995;80(5):1541–1547.

14. Shaw ND, Srouji SS, Histed SN, Hall JE. Differential effects of aging on estrogen negative and positive feedback. *Am J Physiol Endocrinol Metab.* 2011;301(2):E351–E355.

15. O'dea L, Finkelstein JS, Schoenfeld DA, Butler JP, Crowley Jr WF. Interpulse interval of GnRH stimulation independently modulates LH secretion. *Am J Physiol Endocrinol Metab.* 1989;256(4):E510–E515.

16. Couzinet B, Brailly S, Bouchard P, Schaison G. Progesterone stimulates luteinizing hormone secretion by acting directly on the pituitary. *J Clin Endocrinol Metabol.* 1992;74(2):374–378.

17. Welt CK, Pagan YL, Smith PC, Rado KB, Hall JE. Control of follicle-stimulating hormone by estradiol and the inhibins: critical role of estradiol at the hypothalamus during the luteal-follicular transition. *J Clin Endocrinol Metabol.* 2003;88(4):1766–1771.

18. Nippoldt TB, Reame NE, Kelch RP, Marshall JC. The roles of estradiol and progesterone in decreasing luteinizing hormone pulse frequency in the luteal phase of the menstrual cycle. *J Clin Endocrinol Metabol.* 1989;69(1):67–76.

19. Gargett CE, Chan RW, Schwab KE. Endometrial stem cells. *Curr Opin Obstet Gyn.* 2007;19(4):377–383.

20. Figueira PGM, Abrão MS, Krikun G, Taylor H. Stem cells in endometrium and their role in the pathogenesis of endometriosis. *Ann N Y Acad Sci.* 2011;1221(1):10.

21. Slayden OD, Keator CS. Role of progesterone in nonhuman primate implantation. In: *Paper Presented at: Seminars in Reproductive Medicine*; 2007.

22. Wang T, Schneider J. Origin and fate of the nucleolar channel system of normal human endometrium. *Cell Res.* 1992;2(2):97–102.

23. Isaac C, Pollard JW, Meier UT. Intranuclear endoplasmic reticulum induced by Nopp140 mimics the nucleolar channel system of human endometrium. *J Cell Sci.* 2001;114(23):4253–4264.

24. King A. Uterine leukocytes and decidualization. *Hum Reprod Update.* 2000;6(1):28–36.

25. Muñoz-Fernández R, De la Mata C, Prados A, et al. Human predecidual stromal cells have distinctive characteristics of pericytes: cell contractility, chemotactic activity, and expression of pericyte markers and angiogenic factors. *Placenta.* 2018;61:39–47.

26. Aplin J, Charlton A, Ayad S. An immunohistochemical study of human endometrial extracellular matrix during the menstrual cycle and first trimester of pregnancy. *Cell Tissue Res.* 1988;253(1):231–240.

27. Iwahashi M, Muragaki Y, Ooshima A, Yamoto M, Nakano R. Alterations in distribution and composition of the extracellular matrix during decidualization of the human endometrium. *Reproduction.* 1996;108(1):147–155.

28. Salamonsen LA, Lathbury LJ. Endometrial leukocytes and menstruation. *Hum Reprod Update.* 2000;6(1):16–27.

29. Evans J, Salamonsen LA. Inflammation, leukocytes and menstruation. *Rev Endocr Metab Disord.* 2012;13(4):277–288.

30. Curry Jr TE, Osteen KG. The matrix metalloproteinase system: changes, regulation, and impact throughout the ovarian and uterine reproductive cycle. *Endocr Rev.* 2003;24(4):428–465.
31. Cakir M, Mungan I, Karakas T, Girisken I, Okten A. Menstrual pattern and common menstrual disorders among university students in Turkey. *Pediatr Int.* 2007;49(6):938–942.
32. Ju H, Jones M, Mishra G. The prevalence and risk factors of dysmenorrhea. *Epidemiol Rev.* 2014;36(1):104–113.
33. Osayande AS, Mehulic S. Diagnosis and initial management of dysmenorrhea. *Am Fam Physician.* 2014;89(5):341–346.
34. Benjamins LJ, Barratt MS. Evaluation and management of polycystic ovary syndrome. *J Pediatr Health Care.* 2009;23(5):337–343.
35. Albers J, Hull SK, Wesley RM. Abnormal uterine bleeding. *Am Fam Physician.* 2004;69(8):1915–1926.
36. Wiksten-Almströmer M, Hirschberg AL, Hagenfeldt K. Prospective follow-up of menstrual disorders in adolescence and prognostic factors. *Acta Obstet Gynecol Scand.* 2008;87(11):1162–1168.
37. Abdelmoty HI, Youssef M, Abdel-Malak K, et al. Menstrual patterns and disorders among secondary school adolescents in Egypt. A cross-sectional survey. *BMC Women's Health.* 2015;15(1):70.
38. Li X, Feng Y, Lin J-F, Billig H, Shao R. Endometrial progesterone resistance and PCOS. *J Biomed Sci.* 2014;21(1):2.
39. Sen S, Mandal TK, Dutta A, Mondal H, Khalua T. A comparative study of norethisterone and combined oral contraceptive pill in the treatment of dysfunctional uterine bleeding. *CHRISMED J Health Res.* 2019;6(2):87.

Ovarian reserve

4

Zareen Kiran

National Institute of Diabetes and Endocrinology (NIDE), Dow University of Health Sciences (DUHS), Karachi, Pakistan; Section of Endocrinology, Department of Medicine, Aga Khan University Hospital, Karachi, Pakistan

Chapter outline

Introduction

Our concept of human ovarian reserve presumes that the ovary develops several million nongrowing follicles (NGFs) at around 5 months of gestational age. Over the life span of a female, it undergoes a monthly cycle of oocyte maturation as well as integrated endocrine function, which results in a gradual decline of these NGFs. This process continues up to the age of menopause, around 50–51 years, when approximately 1000 NGFs

Subfertility. https://doi.org/10.1016/B978-0-323-75945-8.00004-9

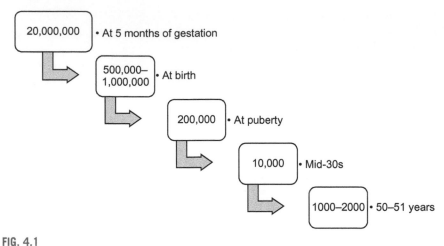

FIG. 4.1

Process showing gradual decline in ovarian follicle pool over different life stages of human ovary.

remain[1,2] (Fig. 4.1). In light of this fact, several biomarkers have evolved to predict as well as evaluate the existing ovarian oocyte pool and foresee the procreative capacity of a human female. More importantly, advanced and assisted reproductive techniques (ARTs) depend heavily upon this background information. Hence, it is a matter of concern to understand the current scientific concepts and available evaluation parameters for ovarian reserve. To make matters even more complex, several hereditary diseases and systemic conditions are associated with decreased ovarian reserve (DOR), which needs to be thoroughly entailed in the clinical situation as well.

Overview of ovarian tissue

Nature has designed ovaries to provide a composite endocrine and reproductive function in a human female. The cascade of events happening during a menstrual cycle is the interplay of various hormones, which help in the fulfillment of these functions. These hormones originate not only from the ovaries but involve the hypothalamus and pituitary gland. However, there are certain autocrine and paracrine factors working alongside the pituitary ovarian axis that have critical roles in reproductive function. These include transforming growth factor-β (TGF-β) family peptides: inhibin A, inhibin B, activin, and the anti-Mullerian hormones.

Histology

A clear description of cortex and medulla in the ovaries is not universally defined, but for functional understanding, cortex includes an area of developing and maturing germ cells, while the medulla is a composition of loose connective tissue. Further details of cortex include surface germinal epithelium, followed by loose mesenchymal cells interspersed between cortical sex cords. This close placement of germ cells and mesangium is meant to provide a well-nurtured and interactive environment for the timely maturation of ovarian follicles. One end of each ovary is designated as the hilum, which aligns the blood vessels and lymphatics to and from the ovaries and provides a surface attachment in the form of mesovarium to the broad ligament.[3,4]

Germ cells

Ovaries are surrounded by a cuboidal germ cell epithelium. This is formed during embryogenesis by the differentiation of somatic cell lineage into primordial germ cells. Several growth factors and ligand interaction lead to the final settlement of these primordial cells on the genital ridge, after which they are referred to as *oogonia*. From there starts the development of primordial follicles with oogonia transforming into mitotic stage *oocytes*. These primordial oocytes then differentiate further into *primary* oocytes within the primary follicles (Fig. 4.2). Finally, any progenitor cell's capability to differentiate into primordial cells is stopped at the stage when oocytes enter into meiosis, and subsequently, further maturation is arrested. This landmark developmental step usually happens around the 8th week of gestation. In reproductive biology, this checkpoint has been conceptualized to mark the final oocyte pool in a human female for her lifetime. However, several experiments over the last decade have negated this concept.[5] On the contrary, clear confirmation about ovarian stem cell reserve and its role in forming an essential component of ovarian reserve is still under development.[6-8]

Endocrine function

After having laid down the essential cellular pillar for human development, it is important to understand its functional chemistry. Several intraovarian paracrine factors and genes take part in the recruitment of early primordial follicles for the developing cohort as detailed in Table 4.1.[9-12]

Stages from primary, secondary, and tertiary follicular growths are therefore follicular-stimulating hormone (FSH)-independent and occur over several menstrual cycles after puberty.[13,14] Maturation of oocytes beyond the meiotic stage comes under the prepubertal FSH effect when each oocyte becomes surrounded by granulosa cell layer. This layer eventually converts into a selected Graafian follicle at the time of puberty when FSH levels are raised in a critical time frame. In each menstrual cycle, the estradiol levels reach their peak near mid-cycle resulting in the complete maturation of a dominant ovarian follicle to mark the process of *ovulation*. But it is only after the luteinizing hormone (LH) surge that ovulation occurs, releasing a mature ovum for fertilization.

The transition of the Graafian follicle to *corpus luteum* after ovulation, a process called *luteinization*, and its sustainability are dependent on the continuous supply of LH or its surrogate human chorionic gonadotropin. The key function

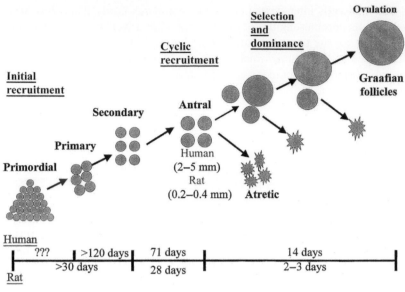

FIG. 4.2

Life history of ovarian follicles. Duration of follicle recruitment and selection in human and rat ovaries. Primordial follicles undergo initial recruitment to enter the growing pool of primary follicles. Due to its protracted nature, the duration required for this step is unknown. In the human ovary, greater than 120 days are required for the primary follicles to reach the secondary follicle stage, whereas 71 days are needed to grow from the secondary to the early antral stage. During cyclic recruitment, increases in circulating FSH allow a cohort of antral follicles (2–5 mm in diameter) to escape apoptotic demise. Among this cohort, a leading follicle emerges as dominant by secreting high levels of estrogens and inhibins to suppress pituitary FSH release. The result is a negative selection of the remaining cohort, leading to its ultimate demise. Concomitantly, increases in local growth factors and vasculature allow a positive selection of the dominant follicle, thus ensuring its final growth and eventual ovulation. After cyclic recruitment, it takes only 2 weeks for an antral follicle to become a dominant Graafian follicle. In rats, the duration of follicle development is much shorter than that needed for human follicles. The time required between the initial recruitment of a primordial follicle and its growth to the secondary stage is more than 30 days, whereas the time for a secondary follicle to reach the early antral stage is about 28 days. Once reaching the early antral stage (0.2–0.4 in diameter), the follicles are subjected to cyclic recruitment, and only 2–3 days are needed for them to grow into preovulatory follicles.

From McGee EA, Hsueh AJ. Initial and cyclic recruitment of ovarian follicles. Endocr Rev. 2000;21(2): 200–214. With permissions: Oxford University Press. Copyright: Oxford University Press.

of constant large production of progesterone from corpus luteum depends on low density lipoprotein (LDL)-cholesterol and functional mitochondrial steroidogenic acute regulatory (STAR) protein.[15] If pregnancy does not take place, then the life of corpus luteum is around 14 days; subsequently, it converts into *corpus albicans.*

Table 4.1 Factors and genes involved in the developmental process of oogenesis.

Paracrine factors	Genes
FIGLA; factor in the germline-α	NOBOX; newborn oogenesis homeobox gene
Foxl2; forkhead box L2	BMP15; bone morphogenetic protein 15 gene
KIT; kit receptor	BRCA1; breast cancer type 1 susceptibility protein gene
KITL; kit ligand	LHCGR; luteinizing hormone/choriogonadotropin receptor gene
IGF; insulin-like growth factor	STAR; steroidogenic acute regulatory protein gene
GDF9; growth differentiation factor 9	CYP11A1; side-chain cleavage enzyme gene
AMH; anti-Mullerian hormone	HSD3B2; 3β-hydroxysteroid dehydrogenase isomerase type 2 gene
NGF; nerve growth factor	CYP17A1; 17-hydroxylase/17,20-lyase gene
BDNF; brain-derived neurotrophic factor	
NT-3 and NT-4; neurotrophin-3 and neurotrophin-4	
GDNF; glial cell line-derived neurotrophic factor	
Inhibin A and inhibin B	
Activin	

Indicators of ovarian reserve
Follicle-stimulating hormone and follicle-stimulating hormone receptors

Gonadotropins belong to the family of peptide hormones with differences in β poly-peptide chains. The FSH is different from other peptide hormones, not only because it is a heterodimer with a different β chain, but it also has different isoforms, which work differently in the normal menstrual cycle.[16] These isoforms are regulated by inhibin B as well as estradiol, which is secreted from granulosa cells inside the growing antral follicle, and are formed in early and late/preovulatory stages of the follicular phase, respectively.[17] The postulation behind this differential activity is to allow maximum follicular growth in the early part of the follicular phase and to enhance more estradiol secretion and therefore support later ovulation. In the context of this hypothesis and its role in follicular growth, there is no doubt that FSH has served as a menopausal as well as ovarian reserve marker for more than a decade.[18,19] However, recent developments in the field of infertility have revealed its clinical utility limitations at least in assessing ovarian oocyte pool and predicting future ART options.[20] More recently, the polymorphisms of genes encoding FSH and FSH receptors have been investigated to show some role in the outcomes of ovarian stimulation therapies and to serve as ovarian reserve markers.[21,22] Although no universal marker is yet completely determined to be sensitive or specific,[23,24] elevated FSH levels continue to be a valuable tool at least in certain clinical settings.[25,26]

Anti-Mullerian hormone and AMH receptor

The anti-Mullerian hormone (AMH), being a glycoprotein, belongs to the TGF-β superfamily. It induces the Mullerian ducts to regress during the male sex differentiation. In cryptorchidic males, it serves as a biochemical marker for testicular tissue.[27] The hormone acts through serine/threonine kinase receptors (AMHRI and AMHRII). The AMH and AMHRII gene defects in men cause one of the conditions of differences of sex differentiation called "persistent Mullerian duct." Recent developments in reproductive medicine have disclosed its role not only on the fetal external genital differentiation but also on the postnatal reproductive life of women. Its levels in women after puberty are similar to those in males and it can serve as an ovarian reserve marker.[28] The granulosa cells of the preantral and small growing follicles are the ovarian sources of AMH.[18,29] It is responsible for the gonadotropin-independent growth of primary follicles and the selection of ovulating follicles from the oocyte pool throughout the lifetime of a human ovary.[30] Particularly, it appears to have a suppressive effect on the collection of primordial follicles and simultaneously stimulates the growing cohort of follicles by increasing their responsiveness to FSH.[31]

From the above discussion, it is clear that AMH is also a reliable prognosticator of time to menopause and is a useful adjunct in the evaluation of a woman's "reproductive age."[32] Besides, higher levels of AMH are associated with a higher count of oocytes or antral follicles retrieved during controlled ovarian stimulation in the in vitro fertilization (IVF) cycles.[13,33] Hence, AMH is also believed as a surrogate marker of the ovarian reserve and is used in pretreatment evaluation of infertile patients for guiding hormonal stimulation.[34,35] Although there is only a slight variation in the AMH level throughout the natural menstrual cycle, optimal timing of measurement during the cycle is still not determined.[36,37] In comparison with other markers described later, AMH was shown to have 100% sensitivity in one of the IVF trials, which assessed markers for poor responders in IVF treatment.[38] Recent reports have also explored the use of AMH in the estimate of ovarian aging in women before or after chemotherapy, predicting the risk of cardiovascular disease near menopause, estimation of long-term reproductive potential following ovarian surgery, in patients with various medical illnesses, and also screening for polycystic ovaries.[39–41] Furthermore, AMH can be used as a biochemical parameter for the diagnosis as well as a tumor marker in therapeutic monitoring for granulosa cell tumors.[34,42]

Inhibin A and inhibin B

Inhibins belong to the members of the broader TGF-β family of autocrine, paracrine, and endocrine factors. Along with other peptide hormones, they are produced by the ovarian granulosa cells under the influence of FSH. While the production of inhibin may occur in many other body tissues including adrenal, pituitary, and placenta, most of it is derived from the gonads. Inhibins have been classified into two heterodimeric isoforms: inhibin A and inhibin B.[43] Their α-subunit is identical, but the β-subunits (βA and βB) are distinct, as they are encoded by separate genes. The main role of inhibins remains to suppress FSH production in the pituitary gland.[17]

Over the past two decades, several useful avenues regarding the inhibin physiology and their clinical significance in reproductive medicine have been discovered.[12] It is now well recognized that the two inhibin isoforms have different secreting patterns during the menstrual cycle.[17] Moreover, inhibins may be involved in the physiological adaptation of pregnancy.[43] Clinically, inhibins may serve as sensitive tumor markers in postmenopausal women, as a useful tool for evaluating ovarian reserve in conditions associated with premature ovarian failure and infertility as well as predicting response to ART.[44,45] Furthermore, inhibins act as a biochemical marker for prenatal screening of Down syndrome as it is a component of the quadruple test, and it also serves in the diagnosis of other feto-maternal disorders.[43,46]

Activin and follistatin

Activin is structurally homologous to inhibin but has functionally reverse actions. Activin is a heterodimer of two subunits that are similar to the β-subunits of inhibins A and B. The three activin isoforms have therefore various combinations of these β-subunits resulting in activin A ($\beta_A\beta_A$), activin B ($\beta_B\beta_B$), and activin AB ($\beta_A\beta_B$). At the pituitary level, activin stimulates the release of FSH, whereas in the ovaries, it augments FSH action. Interestingly, activin is produced in both granulosa cells and pituitary gonadotrophs; however, it is the local activin in the pituitary that regulates the FSH.[43,47]

Follistatin is a monomeric protein produced in the pituitary gland as well as ovaries. It appears to neutralize the biological functions of activin. Therefore, the local follistatin levels in tissues modify the effects of activin. This explains the ultimate suppressive effects that follistatin exerts on pituitary FSH secretion.[43]

The biological role of these TGF-β proteins in determining ovarian reserve as well as other gonadal disorders has been studied for decades but has little development to become clinically applicable.[46,48,49]

Antral follicle count (AFC)

The assessment of the exact number of antral follicles by vaginal ultrasound has long been considered the best test to assess the ovarian reserve and was reviewed in a recent publication.[50] Decreased AFC is one of the major causes of unexplained infertility in a prospective cohort study.[51] In usual practice, on day 3 of the menstrual cycle, a vaginal ultrasound is performed to determine the number of antral follicles.[52] There is no standard definition of an antral follicle. Some investigators considered an antral follicle size between 2 and 5 mm, while others have used the criteria of 10 mm.[53] A review of the literature showed that AFC had a significant positive correlation with levels of serum AMH.[54] An AFC of less than 3–7 indicates a decrease in the ovarian reserve, subsequently reflecting a poor ovarian response to IVF cycles.[55] Recent research has shown a stronger correlation between AFC and oocytes retrieved, as compared to age and FSH levels.[56]

Dynamic ovarian reserve tests

There are several dynamic methods employed in the past to assess ovarian reserve.[57] A quick overview of the steps to conduct these tests is summarized in Table 4.2. Their cumbersome performing methods and technical limitations have rendered them less common in practice.

Clomifene citrate challenge test (CCCT)

Kahraman et al. had reported the sensitivity of CCCT to be 43% and a specificity of 76%, whereas the positive and negative predictive values of this test are 37% and 80%, respectively.[58] The test is performed by checking FSH and estradiol levels on day 3 of the menstrual cycle; then, 100 mg of clomifene citrate is given daily between days 5 and 9 of the cycle, FSH level is then checked again on cycle day 10.[59] With its limitations, it has now become less common in clinical practice.[60] However, it does become part of the assessment of poor (as in primary ovarian insufficiency) and good responders (as in polycystic ovarian syndrome) in ovarian stimulation cycles of IVF.[61]

Exogenous FSH ovarian reserve test (EFORT)

This test comprises cycle day 3 determination of FSH and estradiol levels; thereafter, the patient is given a single injection of FSH 300 IU. On cycle day 4, an estradiol level is checked again. Normal ovarian reserve is defined when the basal FSH is < 11 mIU/mL and the increment in estradiol is > 30 pg/mL. This test first described by Fanchin et al. emphasizes that the synergistic contribution of dynamic change in estradiol and the classically low basal FSH quantities has endorsed the prognostic value of this test.[62] This testing has not been investigated extensively and is not extensively used in the clinical setting due to diagnostic inaccuracy, high cost, and incorrect utility. These limitations revealed in systematic reviews and meta-analysis suggest to abandon them completely.[57,63]

Table 4.2 Dynamic ovarian test methods.

	Step 1	Step 2	Step 3
CCCT	Cycle day 3: FSH and estradiol levels	Cycle days 5 and 9: clomifene citrate 100 mg daily is given	Cycle day 10: FSH level
EFORT	Cycle day 3: FSH and estradiol levels	Single injection of FSH 300 IU given	Cycle day 4: estradiol level
GAST	Cycle day 3: basal FSH, inhibin B, and estradiol levels	A subcutaneous injection of 100 μg triptorelin is given	Cycle day 4: FSH, inhibin B, and estradiol levels

GnRH-agonist stimulation test (GAST)

On cycle day 3, blood is taken for baseline FSH, inhibin B, and estradiol levels, followed by a single subcutaneous injection of 100 μg triptorelin. After 24 h, the same tests are repeated.[64] The analytical precision of GAST, however, could not be determined in several studies due to discrepancies in the way of their performances.[63]

Despite their limited fame, these tests continue to be important in assessing response to gonadotropin treatment in the IVF cycles and remain an important tool in the evaluation of the reproductive potential of a couple.[65]

Disorders affecting ovarian reserve

Genetic abnormalities leading to decreased ovarian reserve (DOR) in females range from significant chromosome abnormalities, submicroscopic chromosome deletion and duplications, and DNA sequence variations in the genes that control numerous biological processes. From the developmental point of view, these processes are implicated in several stages of oogenesis, sustenance of oocyte pool, maintaining a hormonal milieu, and anatomical and functional integrity of female reproductive organs.[66] Moreover, several systemic disorders are associated with early ovarian function decline or defective development from the start.

Chromosomal disorders

1. **Autosomal abnormalities**
   a. **Aneuploidy:** Extra chromosomes on number 13 and 18 have an association with ovarian dysgenesis and failure. Postulating the existence of some ovarian genes to be located on chromosomes 13 and 18, an area requiring further research.[67]
   b. **Autosomal genes:** In otherwise healthy women balanced autosomal translocations have been found resulting in the clinical manifestation of DOR.
   - **Mendelian disorders:** Certain Mendelian disorders are also associated with DOR leading to POI/POF. The list may be evolving; however, some of the common disorders are listed in Table 4.3.[68]
   - **Mitochondrial genes:** Many of the mutated genes that have known to be associated with primary ovarian insufficiency, either isolated or in syndromic cases, also function within mitochondria, including MRPS22, POLG, TWNK, LARS2, HARS2, AARS2, CLPP, and LRPPRC. Collectively, these genes play roles in mitochondrial DNA replication, gene expression, and protein synthesis and degradation.[69] Targeted deletion of mitochondrial fusion protein mitofusin 1 (MFN1) in oocytes resulted in female infertility associated with failure to achieve oocyte maturation. The absence of MFN1 and resulting apoptotic cell loss also caused the depletion of the ovarian

Table 4.3 Mendelian disorders associated with primary ovarian insufficiency/decreased ovarian reserve[a].

Cockayne syndrome
Rothmund–Thomson syndrome
Nijmegen breakage syndrome
Martsolf syndrome
Werner syndrome
Bloom syndrome
ATM gene (ataxia-telangiectasia mental retardation gene)

[a] *For details of each syndrome, see Online Mendelian Inheritance in Man (OMIM).[68]*

follicular reserve, and a phenotype consistent with accelerated female reproductive aging.[70] Low MFN2 expression levels in granulosa cells were related to aging, which may be involved in the clinical outcome of ART by promoting cell apoptosis and affecting mitochondrial function.[71] Caseinolytic peptidase P gene (CLPP) is required for oocyte and embryo development and oocyte mitochondrial function and dynamics. Deficiency of CLPP results in the activation of mTOR pathway, leading to accelerated exhaustion of the ovarian follicular reserve.[72]

- **AMH gene:** Genetically determined age at menarche had no strong association with the levels of AMH. However, genetically determined age at menopause has been linked with lower AMH levels. This concept provides the evidence for genetic support behind the reputable use of AMH as a marker of ovarian reserve.[73]

- **Pigment epithelium-derived factor (PEDF):** Loss of PEDF leads oxidative damage to the ovaries resulting in a diminished ovarian reserve in mice. The mechanism relating this theory is the development of severe insulin resistance and metabolic lipid disorder. PEDF may therefore become a prospective target in the future for the treatment of diseases related to ovarian oxidative damage.[74]

- **BRCA1 and BRCA2 genes:** The mutations of these genes are well known for their association with breast and ovarian cancers. Studies advocate that these patients may also have a risk of low ovarian reserve. Although BRCA mutations are known to alter DNA repair mechanism, it is not proven yet, whether it abates the oocyte ability to mature at least in experimental conditions.[75]

- **Autophagy-related genes:** A study demonstrated that the loss of functions of variant ATG7 and ATG9A genes led to a decrease in autophagosome biosynthesis. This results in a loss of autophagy, which is a crucial biological process required for the process of the preservation of the primordial follicles. Therefore, a functional link is implicated between ATG7 and ATG9A variants and DOR.[76]

- **Micro-RNA expressions:** Previous studies confirmed that micro-RNAs, miR-23a, targets certain protein expressions at the posttranslational level and promote apoptosis in granulosa cells by inhibiting the ERK1/2 signaling pathway.[77,78] Similarly, RNA sequencing (RNA-seq) analysis of human germ cells and corresponding granulosa cells discovered distinctive features. Developmental-stage-specific RNA expression patterns are displayed in the form of several transcriptionally related interactions, machinery, and networks of transcription factors in these cells.[79]
- **Blepharophimosis–ptosis–epicanthus (forkhead transcription factors):** Mutations in the FOXL2 type 1 gene lead to a syndrome of blepharophimosis–ptosis–epicanthus, in almost 70% cases. This is characterized by an autosomal dominant trait; there are abnormalities of the eyelid that co-occur with POF. In specific, the perturbations of forkhead transcription factors cause POI/POF.[80]
- **STAR (steroidogenic acute regulatory) gene:** STAR gene mutations give rise to lipoid congenital adrenal hyperplasia. In later life after puberty, cholesterol accumulation in ovarian cells causes damage, culminating in POI.[81]
- **Perrault syndrome (Connexin 37 gene):** Mutations of Connexin 37 gene leads to what is known as Perrault syndrome, where XX gonadal dysgenesis coexists with sensorineural deafness and inherited in an autosomal recessive disorder.[82]
  - 46, XX gonadal dysgenesis is also reported with certain other genetic syndromes in association with clinical features of cerebellar ataxia, arachnodactyly, and microcephaly, as well as in certain mitochondrial disorders with short stature, and metabolic acidosis.[70]

2. **X Chromosome abnormalities**
   a. **Aneuploidy:** X chromosome aberrations, which include aneuploidies and genetic rearrangements, account for almost 13% of POI cases. **Turner syndrome** is the commonest X chromosomal aneuploidy with a variety of monosomy X (45, X) or mosaicism 45, X/46, XX.[83] Similarly, **triple X syndrome or trisomy X** (47, XXX) is also associated with DOR; however, spontaneous pregnancies are reported.[84]
   b. **Short arms genes**
- **Xp (short arm) genes:** Critical regions on the short arm of the X chromosome (Xp11, Xp22.1–21.3) can be deleted or disrupted. Half of the patients with gonadal dysgenesis in such cases have partial deletions and present with amenorrhea.[85]
- **Zfx (X-linked zinc finger protein):** A widely expressed protein of unknown function is encoded by a gene located on Xp22.1–21.3. Zfx "knockout" progeny of mice are small, subfertile, as they have a reduced germ cell reserve in both gonads.[83,86]

- **USP9X gene (ubiquitin-specific protease 9 gene):** This gene is located on the Xp11.4 region, and its product is extensively expressed in many tissues of the body. In Drosophila, for example, eye development and oogenesis require USP9X gene; however, its function in human gonadal development is still uncertain.[87]
- **Bone morphogenic protein (BMP15):** This gene is located on Xp11.2 and is an essential region for ovarian differentiation. Mutations in this gene had caused primary ovarian insufficiency in American and European Caucasian descent.[88]

c. Long arms genes

- **FMR1 gene:** This is a fragile-X mental retardation 1 gene, found on Xq27.3. Mutations in this gene result in trinucleotide repeat of CGG code in the promoter region of the FMR1 gene.[89] The prevalence of FMR1 gene permutations accounts for approximately 1:150–300 females and 1:400–850 males. This permutation is also associated with the occurrence of a late-onset neurological disorder in male carriers designated as fragile-X tremor ataxia syndrome and several other syndromes like fragile-X-associated primary ovarian insufficiency (FXPOI) and fragile-X-associated diminished ovarian reserve (FXDOR).[90] Why women with the full mutation have no ovarian failure as compared to those with permutation may be linked to random inactivation of the X chromosome.[90]
- **XIST locus (X-inactive specific transcript gene):** The main purpose of this gene product is the revival of the silenced X chromosome during oocyte growth. It is located in the Xq13 region. For normal meiosis to occur, usually two X chromosomes are necessary, in particular with two intact XIST loci. Apoptosis is implicated due to meiotic arrest and oocyte depletion as a result of impaired XIST loci.[85]
- **DIAPH2 gene (diaphanous gene):** Found on Xq21 locus, this gene is identical to the diaphanous gene in Drosophila. The DIA protein is assumed to be important for establishing cell polarity and morphogenesis, and therefore, it is expressed in the ovaries and other tissues in abundance. The disruption of the DIAPH2 gene in Drosophila has shown to cause sterility in both sexes.[91]

Systemic disorders

Several systemic disorders are associated with declining ovarian function either at their start or with the progression of the primary disorder. Moreover, the treatment of certain systemic disorders also leads to declining ovarian function. Clinicians have to keep these conditions in mind while evaluating a patient with decrease ovarian reserve or infertility. Out of some such systemic disorders, as shown in Table 4.4, only a few are described below.

- **Galactose 1–phosphate uridyl transferase (GALT) deficiency:** GALT deficiency results in an inborn error of metabolism called *galactosemia*.

Table 4.4 Systemic disorders affecting ovarian reserve.

Malignant hematologic diseases	Nonmalignant hematologic diseases	Inborn errors of metabolism	Autoimmune diseases
Acute myelogenous leukemia (AML) Chronic myelogenous leukemia (CML) Acute lymphoblastic leukemia (ALL) Chronic lymphocytic leukemia (CLL) Lymphoma: Hodgkin lymphoma Non-Hodgkin lymphoma	Hemoglobinopathies Thalassemia Sickle cell disease Aplastic anemia	Adrenoleukodystrophy Alpha-mannosidosis Aspartylglucosaminidase deficiency Fucosidosis Gaucher disease Hunter syndrome Hurler syndrome Krabbe disease Lysosomal acid lipase deficiency Maroteaux–Lamy syndrome (MPS VI) Morquio syndrome (MPS IV) Mucolipidosis II Sanfilippo syndrome (MPS III) Sly syndrome (MPS VII)	Systemic lupus erythematosus Rheumatoid arthritis (RA) Antiphospholipid syndrome Vasculitis: Behcet's disease (BD) Autoimmune thyroiditis (AIT) Sjögren's syndrome Scleroderma Autoimmune polyglandular syndromes (APS) Myasthenia gravis Multiple sclerosis

Premature ovarian failure may occur in this metabolic disorder along with hypoglycemia and liver dysfunction. The underlying pathology results in biochemical damage to the ovaries.[92]

- **AIRE (autoimmune regulator) gene mutation:** An autoimmune regulator protein expressed in the thymic medulla is encoded by this gene. Mutation of this gene results in a syndrome involving several endocrine organs and ectodermal tissues and is called autoimmune polyendocrinopathy candidiasis-ectodermal dystrophy or autoimmune syndrome type 1. POI occurs due to an autoimmune response to antigens in steroidogenic enzymes and ovarian cells, which culminate in ovarian destruction.[93]

- **Systemic lupus erythematosus (SLE):** Amenorrhea in women with SLE is associated with antibodies against corpus luteum resulting in ovarian failure and raised FSH levels.[94] This has resulted in disease affecting ovarian reserve and future fertility.[95] Besides; patients requiring cyclophosphamide (CYC), an alkylating chemotherapeutic agent has shown to cause POI.[96]

Conclusions

The endocrinology of the human ovaries is a dynamic entity. Decades of dormancy progress into fluctuating secretion of autocrine, paracrine, and hormonal factors until the near-burnout phase of menopause. However, some of the ovarian functioning is assumed to remain even after menopause. "Ovarian reserve testing" assesses this functioning and tells where the ovaries are within this spectrum. Decades ago, a simple endocrine assessment was accepted as the cornerstone of evaluating anovulation and infertility. Rapid advancements in genetics and genome-wide analysis of human DNA have revealed several new etiologies of DOR. Clarifying our understanding of clinical judgment and making the correct diagnosis is an important factor in dealing with a case of an infertile or subfertile couple. Given this, using the right marker of ovarian reserve followed by identifying the correct underlying cause remains a challenge in reproductive endocrinology.

References

1. Faddy M, Gosden R, Gougeon A, Richardson SJ, Nelson JF. Accelerated disappearance of ovarian follicles in mid-life: implications for forecasting menopause. *Hum Reprod.* 1992;7(10):1342–1346.
2. Faddy M, Gosden R. Ovary and ovulation: a model conforming the decline in follicle numbers to the age of menopause in women. *Hum Reprod.* 1996;11(7):1484–1486.
3. Clement PB. Anatomy and histology of the ovary. In: *Blaustein's Pathology of the Female Genital Tract.* Springer; 1987:438–470.
4. Ottolenghi C, Uda M, Hamatani T, et al. Aging of oocyte, ovary, and human reproduction. *Ann NY Acad Sci.* 2004;1034(1):117–131.
5. Li J, Mao Q, He J, She H, Zhang Z, Yin C. Human umbilical cord mesenchymal stem cells improve the reserve function of perimenopausal ovary via a paracrine mechanism. *Stem Cell Res Ther.* 2017;8(1):55.
6. Gheorghisan-Galateanu AA, Hinescu ME, Enciu AM. Ovarian adult stem cells: hope or pitfall? *J Ovarian Res.* 2014;7:71.
7. Sills ES, Wood SH. Autologous activated platelet-rich plasma injection into adult human ovary tissue: molecular mechanism, analysis, and discussion of reproductive response. *Biosci Rep.* 2019;39(6), BSR20190805.
8. Porras-Gomez TJ, Moreno-Mendoza N. Neo-oogenesis in mammals. *Zygote.* 2017;25(4):404–422.
9. Lew R. Natural history of ovarian function including assessment of ovarian reserve and premature ovarian failure. *Best Pract Res Clin Obstet Gynaecol.* 2019;55:2–13.
10. Chang HM, Wu HC, Sun ZG, Lian F, Leung PCK. Neurotrophins and glial cell line-derived neurotrophic factor in the ovary: physiological and pathophysiological implications. *Hum Reprod Update.* 2019;25(2):224–242.
11. Persani L, Rossetti R, Di Pasquale E, Cacciatore C, Fabre S. The fundamental role of bone morphogenetic protein 15 in ovarian function and its involvement in female fertility disorders. *Hum Reprod Update.* 2014;20(6):869–883.
12. Petraglia F, Zanin E, Faletti A, Reis FM. Inhibins: paracrine and endocrine effects in female reproductive function. *Curr Opin Obstet Gynecol.* 1999;11(3):241–247.
13. Edson MA, Nagaraja AK, Matzuk MM. The mammalian ovary from genesis to revelation. *Endocr Rev.* 2009;30(6):624–712.
14. Guzel Y, Oktem O. Understanding follicle growth in vitro: are we getting closer to obtaining mature oocytes from in vitro-grown follicles in human? *Mol Reprod Dev.* 2017;84(7):544–559.

15. Frederick JL, Shimanuki T. Initiation of angiogenesis by human follicular fluid. *Science.* 1984;224(4647):389–390.
16. Andersen CY, Leonardsen L, Ulloa-Aguirre A, Barrios-De-Tomasi J, Moore L, Byskov A. FSH-induced resumption of meiosis in mouse oocytes: effect of different isoforms. *Mol Hum Reprod.* 1999;5(8):726–731.
17. Yding AC. Inhibin-B secretion and FSH isoform distribution may play an integral part of follicular selection in the natural menstrual cycle. *Mol Hum Reprod.* 2017;23(1):16–24.
18. Vural B, Cakiroglu Y, Vural F, Filiz S. Hormonal and functional biomarkers in ovarian response. *Arch Gynecol Obstet.* 2014;289(6):1355–1361.
19. Meden-Vrtovec H. Ovarian aging and infertility. *Clin Exp Obstet Gynecol.* 2004;31(1):5–8.
20. Abdalla H, Thum MY. Repeated testing of basal FSH levels has no predictive value for IVF outcome in women with elevated basal FSH. *Hum Reprod.* 2006;21(1):171–174.
21. La Marca A, Sighinolfi G, Argento C, et al. Polymorphisms in gonadotropin and gonado-tropin receptor genes as markers of ovarian reserve and response in in vitro fertilization. *Fertil Steril.* 2013;99(4). 970–978.e971.
22. Riccetti L, De Pascali F, Gilioli L, et al. Genetics of gonadotropins and their receptors as markers of ovarian reserve and response in controlled ovarian stimulation. *Best Pract Res Clin Obstet Gynaecol.* 2017;44:15–25.
23. van der Steeg JW, Steures P, Eijkemans MJ, et al. Predictive value and clinical impact of basal follicle-stimulating hormone in subfertile, ovulatory women. *J Clin Endocrinol Metab.* 2007;92(6):2163–2168.
24. Haadsma ML, Groen H, Fidler V, et al. The predictive value of ovarian reserve tests for spontaneous pregnancy in subfertile ovulatory women. *Hum Reprod.* 2008;23(8):1800–1807.
25. Singh N, Bahadur A, Malhotra N, Kalaivani M, Mittal S. Prospective analysis of ovarian reserve markers as determinant in response to controlled ovarian stimulation in women undergoing IVF cycles in low resource setting in India. *Arch Gynecol Obstet.* 2013;288(3):697–703.
26. Ayesha, Jha V, Goswami D. Premature ovarian failure: an association with autoimmune diseases. *J Clin Diagn Res.* 2016;10(10):QC10–QC12.
27. Zec I, Tislaric-Medenjak D, Megla ZB, Kucak I. Anti-Mullerian hormone: a unique biochemical marker of gonadal development and fertility in humans. *Biochem Med.* 2011;21(3):219–230.
28. Robeva R, Mekhandzhiev T, Tomova A, Kumanov F. The anti-Mullerian hormone—physiology and application into clinical practice. *Akush Ginekol.* 2006;45(7):50–54.
29. Kedem-Dickman A, Maman E, Yung Y, et al. Anti-Mullerian hormone is highly ex-pressed and secreted from cumulus granulosa cells of stimulated preovulatory immature and atretic oocytes. *Reprod Biomed Online.* 2012;24(5):540–546.
30. Peluso C, Fonseca FL, Rodart IF, et al. AMH: an ovarian reserve biomarker in assisted reproduction. *Clin Chim Acta.* 2014;437:175–182.
31. Shahrokhi SZ, Kazerouni F, Ghaffari F. Anti-Mullerian hormone: genetic and environ-mental effects. *Clin Chim Acta.* 2018;476:123–129.
32. Dolleman M, Depmann M, Eijkemans MJ, et al. Anti-Mullerian hormone is a more ac-curate predictor of individual time to menopause than mother's age at menopause. *Hum Reprod.* 2014;29(3):584–591.
33. Nardo LG, Christodoulou D, Gould D, Roberts SA, Fitzgerald CT, Laing I. Anti-Mullerian hormone levels and antral follicle count in women enrolled in in vitro fertiliza-tion cycles: relationship to lifestyle factors, chronological age and reproductive history. *Gynecol Endocrinol.* 2007;23(8):486–493.

34. Hyldgaard JM, Ingerslev HJ, Torring N, Madsen HN, Bor P. Anti-Mullerian hormone is a clinical useful measure of the ovarian reserve. *Ugeskr Laeger.* 2015;177(5). V09140477.

35. Yates AP, Rustamov O, Roberts SA, et al. Anti-Mullerian hormone-tailored stimulation protocols improve outcomes whilst reducing adverse effects and costs of IVF. *Hum Reprod.* 2011;26(9):2353–2362.

36. Melado L, Lawrenz B, Sibal J, et al. Anti-Mullerian hormone during natural cycle presents significant intra and intercycle variations when measured with fully automated assay. *Front Endocrinol.* 2018;9:686.

37. Gorkem U, Kucukler FK, Togrul C, Gungor T. Anti-Mullerian hormone exhibits a great variation in infertile women with different ovarian reserve patterns. *Aust NZ J Obstet Gynaecol.* 2017;57(4):464–468.

38. Kunt C, Ozaksit G, Keskin Kurt R, et al. Anti-Mullerian hormone is a better marker than inhibin B, follicle stimulating hormone, estradiol or antral follicle count in predicting the outcome of in vitro fertilization. *Arch Gynecol Obstet.* 2011;283(6):1415–1421.

39. Loh JS, Maheshwari A. Anti-Mullerian hormone—is it a crystal ball for predicting ovarian ageing? *Hum Reprod.* 2011;26(11):2925–2932.

40. Broer SL, Broekmans FJ, Laven JS, Fauser BC. Anti-Mullerian hormone: ovarian reserve testing and its potential clinical implications. *Hum Reprod Update.* 2014;20(5):688–701.

41. de Kat AC, Verschuren WM, Eijkemans MJ, Broekmans FJ, van der Schouw YT. Anti-Mullerian hormone trajectories are associated with cardiovascular disease in women: results from the Doetinchem Cohort Study. *Circulation.* 2017;135(6):556–565.

42. Rzeszowska M, Leszcz A, Putowski L, et al. Anti-Mullerian hormone: structure, properties and appliance. *Ginekol Pol.* 2016;87(9):669–674.

43. Makanji Y, Zhu J, Mishra R, et al. Inhibin at 90: from discovery to clinical application, a historical review. *Endocr Rev.* 2014;35(5):747–794.

44. Messina MF, Aversa T, Salzano G, et al. Inhibin B in adolescents and young adults with Turner syndrome. *J Pediatr Endocrinol Metab.* 2015;28(11 − 12):1209–1214.

45. Lockwood G. The diagnostic value of inhibin in infertility evaluation. *Semin Reprod Med.* 2004;22(3):195–208.

46. Robertson DM. Inhibins and activins in blood: predictors of female reproductive health? *Mol Cell Endocrinol.* 2012;359(1–2):78–84.

47. Seachrist DD, Keri RA. The activin social network: activin, inhibin, and follistatin in breast development and cancer. *Endocrinology.* 2019;160(5):1097–1110.

48. Pangas SA. Regulation of the ovarian reserve by members of the transforming growth factor beta family. *Mol Reprod Dev.* 2012;79(10):666–679.

49. Lahlou N, Bouvattier C, Linglart A, Rodrigue D, Teinturier C. The role of gonadal peptides in clinical investigation. *Ann Biol Clin.* 2009;67(3):283–292.

50. Khan HL, Bhatti S, Suhail S, et al. Antral follicle count (AFC) and serum anti-Mullerian hormone (AMH) are the predictors of natural fecundability have similar trends irrespective of fertility status and menstrual characteristics among fertile and infertile women below the age of 40 years. *Reprod Biol Endocrinol.* 2019;17(1):20.

51. Yucel B, Kelekci S, Demirel E. Decline in ovarian reserve may be an undiagnosed reason for unexplained infertility: a cohort study. *Arch Med Sci.* 2018;14(3):527–531.

52. Xu H, Zeng L, Yang R, Feng Y, Li R, Qiao J. Retrospective cohort study: AMH is the best ovarian reserve markers in predicting ovarian response but has unfavorable value in predicting clinical pregnancy in GnRH antagonist protocol. *Arch Gynecol Obstet.* 2017;295(3):763–770.

53. Broekmans FJ, de Ziegler D, Howles CM, Gougeon A, Trew G, Olivennes F. The antral follicle count: practical recommendations for better standardization. *Fertil Steril.* 2010;94(3):1044–1051.

54. Bhide P, Pundir J, Homburg R, Acharya G. Biomarkers of ovarian reserve in childhood and adolescence: a systematic review. *Acta Obstet Gynecol Scand.* 2019;98(5):563–572.

55. Himabindu Y, Sriharibabu M, Gopinathan K, Satish U, Louis TF, Gopinath P. Anti-Mullerian hormone and antral follicle count as predictors of ovarian response in assisted reproduction. *J Human Reprod Sci.* 2013;6(1):27.

56. Siddiqui QUA, Anjum S, Zahra F, Yousuf SM. Ovarian reserve parameters and response to controlled ovarian stimulation in infertile patients. *Pak J Med Sci.* 2019;35(4):958–962.

57. La Marca A, Argento C, Sighinolfi G, et al. Possibilities and limits of ovarian reserve testing in ART. *Curr Pharm Biotechnol.* 2012;13(3):398–408.

58. Kahraman S, Vicdan K, Isik AZ, et al. Clomiphene citrate challenge test in the assessment of ovarian reserve before controlled ovarian hyperstimulation for intracytoplasmic sperm injection. *Eur J Obstet Gynecol Reprod Biol.* 1997;73(2):177–182.

59. Scott RT, Leonardi MR, Hofmann GE, Illions EH, Neal GS, Navot D. A prospective evaluation of clomiphene citrate challenge test screening of the general infertility population. *Obstet Gynecol.* 1993;82(4 pt 1):539–544.

60. Broer Simone L, van Disseldorp Jeroen, Broeze Kimiko A, et al., IMPORT study group. Added value of ovarian reserve testing on patient characteristics in the prediction of ovarian response and ongoing pregnancy: an individual patient data approach. Hum. Reprod. Update. 19(1):26–36. 1460-2369. doi:10.1093/humupd/dms041. 23188168.

61. Kwee J, Schats R, McDonnell J, Schoemaker J, Lambalk CB. The clomiphene citrate challenge test versus the exogenous follicle-stimulating hormone ovarian reserve test as a single test for identification of low responders and hyperresponders to in vitro fertilization. *Fertil Steril.* 2006;85(6):1714–1722.

62. Fanchin R, de Ziegler D, Olivennes F, Taieb J, Dzik A, Frydman R. Endocrinology: exogenous follicle stimulating hormone ovarian reserve test (EFORT): a simple and reliable screening test for detecting 'poor responders' in in-vitro fertilization. *Hum Reprod.* 1994;9(9):1607–1611.

63. Maheshwari A, Gibreel A, Bhattacharya S, Johnson NP. Dynamic tests of ovarian reserve: a systematic review of diagnostic accuracy. *Reprod Biomed Online.* 2009;18(5):717–734.

64. Hendriks D, Broekmans F, Bancsi L, Looman C, De Jong F, Te Velde E. Single and repeated GnRH agonist stimulation tests compared with basal markers of ovarian reserve in the prediction of outcome in IVF. *J Assist Reprod Genet.* 2005;22(2):65–74.

65. Sills ES, Alper MM, Walsh AP. Ovarian reserve screening in infertility: practical applications and theoretical directions for research. *Eur J Obstet Gynecol Reprod Biol.* 2009;146(1):30–36.

66. Yatsenko SA, Rajkovic A. Genetics of human female infertility. *Biol Reprod.* 2019;101(3):549–566.

67. Grande M, Borobio V, Bennasar M, et al. Role of ovarian reserve markers, antimullerian hormone and antral follicle count, as aneuploidy markers in ongoing pregnancies and miscarriages. *Fertil Steril.* 2015;103(5):1221–1227. e1222.

68. Hamosh A, Scott AF, Amberger JS, Bocchini CA, McKusick VA. Online Mendelian Inheritance in Man (OMIM), a knowledgebase of human genes and genetic disorders. *Nucleic Acids Res.* 2005;33(suppl. 1). D514–D517.

69. Tiosano D, Mears JA, Buchner DA. Mitochondrial dysfunction in primary ovarian insufficiency. *Endocrinology.* 2019;160(10):2353–2366.

70. Zhang M, Bener MB, Jiang Z, et al. Mitofusin 1 is required for female fertility and to maintain ovarian follicular reserve. *Cell Death Dis.* 2019;10(8):560.

71. Wang L, Song S, Liu X, Zhang M, Xiang W. Low MFN2 expression related to ageing in granulosa cells is associated with assisted reproductive technology outcome. *Reprod Biomed Online.* 2019;38(2):152–158.

72. Wang T, Babayev E, Jiang Z, et al. Mitochondrial unfolded protein response gene Clpp is required to maintain ovarian follicular reserve during aging, for oocyte competence, and development of pre-implantation embryos. *Aging Cell.* 2018;17(4), e12784.

73. Ruth KS, Soares ALG, Borges MC, et al. Genome-wide association study of anti-Mullerian hormone levels in pre-menopausal women of late reproductive age and relationship with genetic determinants of reproductive lifespan. *Hum Mol Genet.* 2019;28(8):1392–1401.

74. Li XH, Wang HP, Tan J, et al. Loss of pigment epithelium-derived factor leads to ovarian oxidative damage accompanied by diminished ovarian reserve in mice. *Life Sci.* 2019;216:129–139.

75. Grynberg M, Dagher Hayeck B, Papanikolaou EG, Sifer C, Sermondade N, Sonigo C. BRCA1/2 gene mutations do not affect the capacity of oocytes from breast cancer candidates for fertility preservation to mature in vitro. *Hum Reprod.* 2019;34(2):374–379.

76. Delcour C, Amazit L, Patino LC, et al. ATG7 and ATG9A loss-of-function variants trigger autophagy impairment and ovarian failure. *Genet Med.* 2019;21(4):930–938.

77. Luo H, Han Y, Liu J, Zhang Y. Identification of microRNAs in granulosa cells from patients with different levels of ovarian reserve function and the potential regulatory function of miR-23a in granulosa cell apoptosis. *Gene.* 2019;686:250–260.

78. Woo I, Christenson LK, Gunewardena S, et al. Micro-RNAs involved in cellular proliferation have altered expression profiles in granulosa of young women with diminished ovarian reserve. *J Assist Reprod Genet.* 2018;35(10):1777–1786.

79. Zhang Y, Yan Z, Qin Q, et al. Transcriptome landscape of human folliculogenesis reveals oocyte and granulosa cell interactions. *Mol Cell.* 2018;72(6):1021–1034. e1024.

80. Bertini V, Valetto A, Baldinotti F, et al. Blepharophimosis, ptosis, epicanthus inversus syndrome: new report with a 197-kb deletion upstream of FOXL2 and review of the literature. *Mol Syndromol.* 2019;10(3):147–153.

81. Bhangoo A, Buyuk E, Oktay K, Ten S. Phenotypic features of 46, XX females with StAR protein mutations. *Pediatr Endocrinol Rev.* 2007;5(2):633–641.

82. Simon AM, Goodenough DA, Li E, Paul DL. Female infertility in mice lacking connexin 37. *Nature.* 1997;385(6616):525.

83. Fortuno C, Labarta E. Genetics of primary ovarian insufficiency: a review. *J Assist Reprod Genet.* 2014;31(12):1573–1585.

84. Otter M, Schrander-Stumpel CT, Curfs LM. Triple X syndrome: a review of the literature. *Eur J Hum Genet.* 2010;18(3):265.

85. Simpson JL. Genetic and phenotypic heterogeneity in ovarian failure: overview of selected candidate genes. *Ann NY Acad Sci.* 2008;1135(1):146–154.

86. Luoh S-W, Bain PA, Polakiewicz RD, et al. Zfx mutation results in small animal size and reduced germ cell number in male and female mice. *Development.* 1997;124(11):2275–2284.

87. Simpson JL, Rajkovic A. Ovarian differentiation and gonadal failure. *Am J Med Genet.* 1999;89(4):186–200.

88. Di Pasquale E, Beck-Peccoz P, Persani L. Hypergonadotropic ovarian failure associated with an inherited mutation of human bone morphogenetic protein-15 (BMP15) gene. *Am J Hum Genet*. 2004;75(1):106–111.

89. Wittenberger MD, Hagerman RJ, Sherman SL, et al. The FMR1 premutation and reproduction. *Fertil Steril*. 2007;87(3):456–465.

90. Man L, Lekovich J, Rosenwaks Z, Gerhardt J. Fragile X-associated diminished ovarian reserve and primary ovarian insufficiency from molecular mechanisms to clinical manifestations. *Front Mol Neurosci*. 2017;10:290.

91. Bione S, Sala C, Manzini C, et al. A human homologue of the Drosophila melanogaster diaphanous gene is disrupted in a patient with premature ovarian failure: evidence for conserved function in oogenesis and implications for human sterility. *Am J Hum Genet*. 1998;62(3):533–541.

92. Spencer JB, Badik JR, Ryan EL, et al. Modifiers of ovarian function in girls and women with classic galactosemia. *J Clin Endocrinol Metab*. 2013;98(7):E1257–E1265.

93. Fierabracci A, Bizzarri C, Palma A, Milillo A, Bellacchio E, Cappa M. A novel heterozygous mutation of the AIRE gene in a patient with autoimmune polyendocrinopathy-candidiasis-ectodermal dystrophy syndrome (APECED). *Gene*. 2012;511(1):113–117.

94. Pasoto S, Viana V, Mendonca B, Yoshinari N, Bonfa E. Anti-corpus luteum antibody: a novel serological marker for ovarian dysfunction in systemic lupus erythematosus? *J Rheumatol*. 1999;26(5):1087–1093.

95. Di Mario C, Petricca L, Gigante MR, et al. Correction to: Anti-Mullerian hormone serum levels in systemic lupus erythematosus patients: influence of the disease severity and therapy on the ovarian reserve. *Endocrine*. 2019;63(2):405.

96. Mersereau J, Dooley MA. Gonadal failure with cyclophosphamide therapy for lupus nephritis: advances in fertility preservation. *Rheum Dis Clin North Am*. 2010;36(1):99–108. viii.

Introduction to subfertility

5

Faiza Alam

Clinical Academia, Pengiran Anak Puteri Rashidah Sa'adatul Bolkiah Institute of Health Science, Universiti Brunei Darussalam, Bandar Seri Begawan, Brunei

Chapter outline

Having babies is a right and wish of all the couples after marriage, but an intact hormonal system, psychological stability, and emotional composure are the merits for achieving due to maturation of the sperm and ovum leading to the fertilization followed by the birth of a healthy being. Fertility refers to the ability to conceive and bear offsprings, while fecundity expresses the prospect of women to reproduce on a monthly basis.[1] The incompetence of a couple to conceive after more than 12 months of unprotected intercourse is

Subfertility. https://doi.org/10.1016/B978-0-323-75945-8.00005-0

called "infertility." According to the World Health Organization, "infertility is the inability to conceive a child." Inability of a woman to become pregnant after 1 year of regular intercourse for what so ever the cause may be labels the couple as infertile.[2]

Infertility is consistent with all cultures and societies and affects an estimated 10%–15% of couples of reproductive age worldwide.[3] Every one in six couples is affected by this debarment. Infertility is prevalent in all societies of the world, including 50% of West African societies, 12% of Western European families, and 23% of couples in Pakistan. This universal burden is growing at a tremendous rate with topographical variations and affecting the quality of life of not only the married couples but also families at large. It is undoubtedly a key threat to a married female and demands financial stability for its investigation and choice of treatment plans eventually.

Prevalence

Infertility is taken as a problem in every culture and society and is considered to affect approximately 10%–15% of couples of reproductive ages. Lately, the graph of treatment-seeking couples for infertility has gone high due to many factors including delayed marriages, belated childbearing in women, and knowledge of the development of successful new techniques for infertility treatment.

Infertility can be classified as "primary infertility," a condition where the female is deprived of conceiving at all or has been unable to carry on pregnancy fruitfully to a live birth, and "secondary infertility," where the female is incapable of conceiving a new pregnancy for 1 year following a previous pregnancy. Primary infertility contributes 5% of the 23% infertile couples while secondary type of infertility is approximately three times more.[4]

According to WHO-DHS Comparative Report, 2004, approximately 186 million women of the developing countries (excluding China) are suffering from any type of infertility.[5] This number represents that in every four ever-married women, more than one woman is subfertile during their reproductive age. The prevalence of infertility in Pakistan is approximately 23%, where primary infertility contributes to 3.5%–3.9% and secondary infertility is 18.0%–18.4%.[6]

Determinants of male subfertility

Men and women are **equally (40%)** responsible for infertility while the remaining 20% couples have no identified cause for conception (unexplained infertility).[7] Apart from physiological variations, three types of factors can act by themselves or interact in complex pathways, which are environmental, genetic, and physiological. The causes are summarized in Fig. 5.1.

Known etiology of male factor subfertility is around 10% and repeated specimen analysis of semen can reduce this rate to 2%. The normal values of semen characteristics are given in the previous chapter.

Male infertility contributes to 40% of the total cases of subfertility. Abnormal semen characteristics have no reason (idiopathic) in around 26% of infertile men.

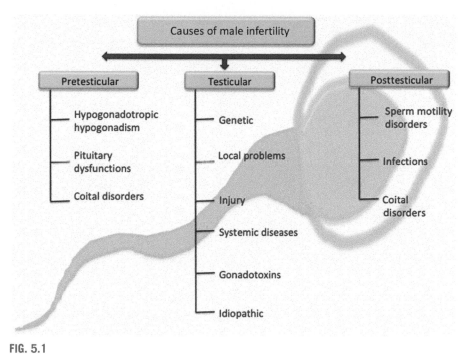

FIG. 5.1

Causes of male infertility.

Oligoasthenoteratozoospermia is characterized by dysfunctional spermatozoa, whereby some percentage of sperms is incapable of fertilization. Antisperm antibodies are a probable cause of this condition.[8]

Hypothalamic pituitary failure may lead to azoospermia. Its two types are nonobstructive azoospermia causing primary testicular failure and obstructive azoospermia causing the obstruction of the genital tract.

Less than 1% of the infertile men problems are due to hypothalamic or pituitary dysfunctions. In this case, luteinizing hormone and follicular-stimulating hormone are less than normal, which affects the normal spermatogenesis and testosterone production and secretion.

Causes of female subfertility

In general, the causes or factors of female infertility can be classified based on whether they are acquired or genetic, or strictly on the basis of location. Causes of infertility in the Pakistani population can broadly be categorized into male factors (23%), female (44%) or unexplained infertility (28%), and coital factors (5%).

A number of dietary, infectious, environmental, endocrine as well as hormonal imbalances can be the contributing factors. Hence, female infertility turns out to be

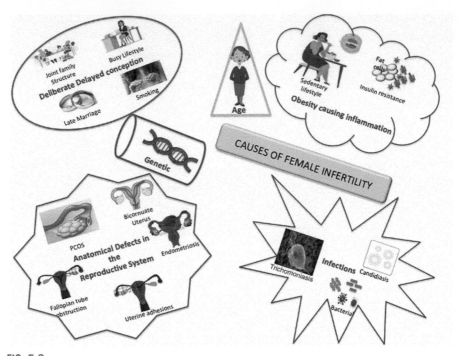

FIG. 5.2

Potential factors affecting female fertility.

a pressing global burden, especially in South Asian countries. It is a well-known fact that the scale of infertility spreads from the reproductive disorders leading to detrimental psychological as well as social implications[9–11] (Fig. 5.2).

Delayed conception

The known causes of infertility are mostly related to defects in fallopian tubes, uterus, or hormonal balance. The increase in age at the time of marriage due to the attainment of higher education is another contributing factor. Increased age (>35 years) affects the efficiency of ovaries and has been documented to be reciprocal with reproductive capacity.[12] Additionally, females being work-oriented and pursuing professional growth tend to spend hours at a job, and later, being tired has also decreased the frequency of sexual intercourse and increased the chromosomal abnormalities and rate of abortions.[11]

Lifestyle

Apart from physiological aspects, the occupation of the couple is another point of concern. Long working hours or shift duties may affect the frequency and correct timings of sexual intercourse. Exposure to radiations, harmful substances, and heat is likely to reduce sperm parameters in males. Living in a joint family system with the burden of household chores makes workingwomen too tired to be available to male partners. Monitoring the body basal temperature or maintaining a monthly chart of the menstrual cycle could be helpful in achieving conception by coinciding with ovulation.[13]

The consumption of alcohol has not been effectively found to be associated with female infertility, but excessive alcohol intake has reversible detrimental effects on sperm quality. However, smoking has a strong association with delayed conception, reducing infertility in females and with derangement of sperm parameters in males.[14] There is no consistent evidence to demonstrate an association between caffeinated drinks and fertility difficulties.

Obesity

Obesity stands as a well-known independent risk factor for not only cardiovascular diseases and diabetes mellitus but also reproductive malfunction in both males and females and has been associated with lower success rates following assisted reproduction.[15] Integral differences òf oocytes in these obese patients increase with the duration of stimulation, decrease number of oocytes, and affect oocyte maturity, implantation, and clinical pregnancy rates.[16] Obesity impacts females starting from menstrual irregularities to delayed conception and spontaneous abortions in females; obesity has a negative association with erectile function and normal amount motile sperms.

Endometriosis

Endometriosis is a term given to a condition where the endometrial tissue is found outside the uterine cavity. It accounts for 5% of female infertility and is characterized by peritoneal lesions, adhesions, and cysts. Mild endometriosis is equivalent to unexplained infertility in females.

Anatomical defects

Uterine abnormalities include uterine or cervical polyps, submucosal leiomyomas, and adhesions within the reproductive tract. Bicornuate uterus is also a contributor to female infertility. The reason for this association has to be elucidated.

Infections

Gonorrhea, tuberculosis, and chlamydiasis are the most common causes of infection of the female reproductive tract. During infection, the tubal lining is damaged, which later causes adhesions that interfere with the normal ovum transport to the appropriate site of fertilization and implantation. These sequelae may result in ectopic pregnancy, abscesses, pelvic inflammatory diseases, and hydrosalpinx. Infections from chlamydia trachomatis range from 11% to 13% in the young population. It stands as a major cause of pelvic inflammatory disease resulting in abdominal pain, ectopic pregnancies, or infertility due to tubal incompetence. Routine uterine investigations for infertility, including cervical hysterosalpingography, might extend or reactivate the infection. Cervical cancers have also been reported as the cause of delayed fertility.[17]

Genetic trait of subfertility

Chromosomal aberrations and gene variation are common causes of infertility. Obesity being a part of PCOs suggests that genes responsible for causing PCOs are employed in reproductive hormone regulation, steroid biosynthesis, and insulin sensitization. Calcium dependency for egg activation, oocyte maturation, follicular growth, and embryo development involves the vitamin D receptor genetic mutations to be associated with PCOs. Apart from genes directly involved in reproductive hormones, mitochondrial genes have also been associated with female infertility.

Unexplained subfertility

Unexplained subfertility is a term used when a couple is incapable of conceiving with no detachable cause. It includes 40% of the infertile females and about 8%–28% of the infertile couples, worldwide.

Oxidative stress

A lot of research is focused on the evaluation of oxidative stress as a cause of infertility in females. Evidence proves the presence of altered redox environment in the sperms and the seminal fluid; however, the evaluation of oxidative disturbances in the granulosa cells and the follicular fluid needs to be investigated in depth. Occupation, long working hours, and presence of emotional stress on the infertile females play a major role in developing this condition, which becomes one more factor for unsuccessful attempts to assisted reproductive techniques (ART).[11] Details of ART are discussed in Chapter 6.

Current methods employed for investigating subfertility and challenges faced in clinical practice

Assessment of male factor infertility

- Semen analysis
  As per the guideline development group, the sperm analysis criteria set by the WHO for the detection of male factor infertility are not specific but sensitive; thus, semen specimen should be retested two to three times to reduce false-positive cases.

- Antisperm antibody
- Hypothalamic pituitary failure (nonobstructive) and patency of the genital tract (nonobstructive) should be examined in the case of azoospermia.
- Cervical mucus postcoital testing (PCT): As per the evidence, there is no effect of the PCT on the treatment strategies.[18]

Assessment of ovarian disorders

- Evaluating ovarian reserves
  The fertility of a woman is directly proportional to its ovarian reserve. With an increase in age, the reserve declines and thus decreases the probability of becoming pregnant. Apart from age, the hormonal levels are very important determinants of the ovarian reserve. Antral follicle count (AFC), anti-Mullerian hormone (AMH), follicle stimulating hormone (FSH), and clomifene citrate challenge are recognized to fulfill the accuracy criteria for detecting the ovarian reserve. However, after analysis, these tests are unable to predict live birth accurately. Live birth is the most important and desirable outcome from all tests and treatments thus demands determination of accurate cutoffs for its prediction.
- Regularity of menstrual cycle
  The cycle ranging from 26 to 39 days is considered as a normal regulation of menstrual cycle. It is characterized by the luteinizing hormone (LH) surge, which can be detected by monitoring basal body temperature. Urinary LH kits are also helpful in identifying forthcoming ovulation. Mid-luteal progesterone levels around 21st day are also indicative of ovulation but are very nonspecific in females with irregular cycles.
- Thyroid function test
  Screening infertile females for thyroid function has been a routine, as hypothyroidism is known for causing disturbed menstrual and anovulatory cycles.

Tubal and uterine disorders

- Hysterosalpingography vs laparoscopy with dye
  Both invasive procedures are widely used to detect the patency of the ovarian tubes, where they identify tubal blockade as a cause of infertility they show no reliability for positive pregnancy outcomes.
  Laparoscopy stands as a gold standard for uterine pathologies; however, HSG records the patency.
- Falloposcopy
  This transvaginal microendoscopy approach is well recognized for the detection of the entire fallopian tube patency. Furthermore, studies show that 24% of females conceived naturally after this procedure.[19]
- Tubal flushing
  Tubal flushing showed a significant increase in pregnancy rate when performed with oil-soluble contrast. However, further studies to assess the effect of

water-soluble media on the pregnancy rate and outcome are warranted. Anaphylaxis and lipogranuloma have been reported to occur as a consequence of this tubal patency testing.
- Ultrasound of pelvis
  Still standing as the first-most line of investigation to rule out pelvic pathologies, ultrasound pelvis provides great accuracy and reliability.

Treating infections

- Various techniques are used to reduce the transmission of sexually transmitted diseases depending on the virus under the suspect. An approach like sperm washing is used to prevent hepatitis C while hepatitis B can be prevented via vaccines. In vitro fertilization (IVF) and intracytoplasmic sperm injection (ICSI) play a great role in prevention from human immunodeficiency virus (HIV) as this technique provides a washed sperm preparation. However, sperm washing does not guarantee the complete elimination of the virus.
- Less invasive and more cost-effective treatment ways include antiviral therapy for couples where one partner is HIV-positive.

Role of Chinese herbal medicine for treating PCOS

- PCOS is a combination of obesity, insulin resistance, and hyperlipidemia; thus, a true picture of metabolic syndrome patients. Chinese herbal medicine (CHM) is widely used for various metabolic dysfunctions involving kidneys, heart, and liver. It is also used in treating menstrual disorders, hirsutism, and improving pregnancy rate in PCOS patients.
- Routinely CHM is considered as a safe regimen provided prescribed appropriately by qualified practitioners. There are serious concerns about unfavorable incidents, including allergic reactions and kidney involvement like Chinese herbal nephropathy (CHN) [20–22]. Utilization of this type of therapy needs a detailed research before labeling it reliable.

Evaluation of genetic problems

- Before finalizing the treatment of subfertility in both males and females, genetic defects should be considered and discussed in detail with the couple in order to be explicit about the outcomes. Karyotyping should become a routine investigation, especially in infertile males with deformed sperms and nonobstructive azoospermia. Microdeletion of Y chromosome is not very common and thus not regarded as a part of routine investigation.
- ICSI and IVF are popular choices of infertility treatment. ICSI has a better fertilization rate; however, pregnancy rate is observed to be better after IVF.

References

1. Wood JW. Fecundity and natural fertility in humans. *Oxf Rev Reprod Biol.* 1989;11:61–109.
2. Agarwal A, Majzoub A. Role of antioxidants in assisted reproductive techniques. *World J Mens Health.* 2017;35(2):77–93.
3. Cui W. *Mother or Nothing: The Agony of Infertility.* SciELO Public Health; 2010.
4. Sami N, Ali TS, Wasim S, Saleem S. Risk factors for secondary infertility among women in Karachi, Pakistan. *PLoS One.* 2012;7(4), e35828.
5. Ali S, Sophie R, Imam AM, et al. Knowledge, perceptions and myths regarding infertility among selected adult population in Pakistan: a cross-sectional study. *BMC Public Health.* 2011;11(1):760.
6. Shaheen R, Fazil S, Sultan S, Subhan K, Tahir F. Prevalence of infertility in a cross section of Pakistani population. *Pak J Zool.* 2010;42(4):389–393.
7. Agarwal A, Mulgund A, Hamada A, Chyatte MR. A unique view on male infertility around the globe. *Reprod Biol Endocrinol.* 2015;13:37. https://doi.org/10.1186/s12958-015-0032-1.
8. Xu YC, Jing LI, Liang WB, Zhu WJ. Evaluation on antisperm antibody in infertile men with oligoasthenoteratozoospermia. *J Reprod Contracept.* 2014;25:49–53.
9. Mumtaz A, Khalid A, Jamil Z, Fatima SS, Arif S, Rehman R. Kisspeptin: a potential factor for unexplained infertility and impaired embryo implantation. *Int J Fert Ster.* 2017;11(2):99.
10. Tarín JJ, García-Pérez MA, Hamatani T, Cano A. Infertility etiologies are genetically and clinically linked with other diseases in single meta-diseases. *Reprod Biol Endocrinol.* 2015;13:31. https://doi.org/10.1186/s12958-015-0029-9.
11. Alam F, Khan TA, Rehman R. Stress of infertility: can the couple cope? *JPMA.* 2018;68(4):679–680.
12. Rehman R, Fatima SS, Alam F, Ashraf M, Zafar S. Kisspeptin and attributes of infertile males and females: a cross sectional study in a subset of Pakistani population. *Andrologia.* 2019;51(9), e13370. https://doi.org/10.1111/and.13370.
13. Su HW, Yi YC, Wei TY, Chang TC, Cheng CM. Detection of ovulation, a review of currently available methods. *Bioeng Transl Med.* 2017;2(3):238–246. https://doi.org/10.1002/btm2.10058.
14. Rehman R, Zahid N, Amjad S, Baig M, Gazzaz ZJ. Relationship between smoking habit and sperm parameters among patients attending an infertility clinic. *Front Physiol.* 2019;10:1356. https://doi.org/10.3389/fphys.2019.01356.
15. Fedorcsak P, Dale PO, Storeng R, et al. Impact of overweight and underweight on assisted reproduction treatment. *Hum Reprod.* 2004;19(11):2523–2528.
16. Spandorfer SD, Kump L, Goldschlag D, Brodkin T, Davis OK, Rosenwaks Z. Obesity and in vitro fertilization: negative influences on outcome. *J Reprod Med.* 2004;49(12):973–977.
17. Karim S, Souho T, Benlemlih M, Bennani B. Cervical cancer induction enhancement potential of chlamydia trachomatis: a systematic review. *Curr Microbiol.* 2018;75(12):1667–1674. https://doi.org/10.1007/s00284-018-1439-7.
18. Balasch J. Investigation of the infertile couple in the era of assisted reproductive technology: a time for reappraisal. *Hum Reprod.* 2000;15:2251–2257.
19. Downing BG, Wood C. Predictive value of falloscopy: 200 case study. *Ref Gynecol Obstet.* 1995;3:156–162.

20. Nortier JL, Martinez MC, Schmeiser HH, Arlt VM, Bieler CA, Petein M. Urothelial carcinoma associated with the use of a Chinese herb (*Aristolochia fangchi*). *N Eng J Med.* 2000;342(23):1686–1692.
21. Lord GM, Cook T, Arlt VM, Schmeiser HH, Williams G, Pusey CD. Urothelial malignant disease and Chinese herbal nephropathy. *Lancet.* 2001;358(9292):1515–1516.
22. Lampert N, Xu Y. Chinese herbal nephropathy. *Lancet.* 2002;359(9308):796–797.

Impact of subfertility

6

Faiza Alam

Clinical Academia, Pengiran Anak Puteri Rashidah Sa'adatul Bolkiah Institute of Health Science, Universiti Brunei Darussalam, Bandar Seri Begawan, Brunei

Chapter outline

Impact of subfertility

Irrespective of the society, culture, class, division, and educational status of an individual, subfertility effects both the male and the female. Both have an equal sense of the debarment; nevertheless, it has been observed that for various reasons in different cultures, females are stigmatized for being responsible for this condition. Influence of infertility has resulted in the aggravation of medial, social, psychological, and economic burdens of developing countries.[1] Infertile couples receive discriminative treatment from society, especially from friends and relatives. Our culture imposes social pressure more on newly married women in this context, especially to have sons. The debarment places infertile women in a lonely place shadowed by pain, agony, sorrow, and empathy.[2] Various losses faced by infertile couples may include loss of health, self-esteem, self-assurance, parental identity, personal control, genetic legacy, grand-parenting relationship, trust in religion, optimism in the future, sexual identity, and childbearing and child-rearing experience in the long list of deprivations for the infertile couples.[2] Commonly, infertile females of the Third World countries feel profound self-reproach and embarrassment for this condition. Generally, the impact of infertility can broadly be characterized into physical, social, psychological, and economic factors.

Subfertility. https://doi.org/10.1016/B978-0-323-75945-8.00006-2

Effect on the marital relationship

A number of infertile females regret to accept that during their struggle with subfertility, their relationship with their husbands has been negatively affected. Stress-related alteration of the hypothalamic–pituitary–adrenal (HPA) axis influences the human pituitary ovarian (HPO) axis, which results in the modified sexual behavior along with changes in the luteinizing hormone-releasing hormone and luteinizing hormone levels. Increased levels of cortisol and proopiomelanocortin (POMC) reduce the synthesis of sex hormones accounting for the changes in the HPA and HPO axis, which along with other hormones affects the release of oxytocin. Oxytocin is also involved in the maintenance of social and sexual life. Evidence shows that adequate levels of oxytocin keep the mood and sexual drive of a female elevated; however, it modulates the transport of the sperm within the female genital tract.

Many a times the psychological irritability going on within the woman's mind, the burden of treatment, its schedule, and the finances involved in this process make the marriage stressful. It has been observed that some men are against the infertility investigation and treatments as; (i) they are petrified of being responsible for the cause (male infertility), a big taboo on manhood!, (ii) it comes with financial burden (especially for the rural dwellers), (iii) they do not want to miss the chance of second marriage, (iv) they are unaware of the treatment success rate and its impact, (v) they are too busy to actually feel the debarment, and (vi) the believe it collides with their social and religious beliefs. In some scenarios, the man demands child but females are either: (i) not willing for the treatment and (ii) too career-oriented and feel that an additional responsibility of becoming pregnant and bearing a child might hinder their success. Whatever the reason, subfertility leads to arguments and eventually affects the marital relationship.

Psychological effects

The feeling of losing their "womanhood" renders the women not to be considered as a "woman" if they do not have a child. A newlywed female faces a great social pressure, to conceive on as soon as possible basis, which becomes a psychological burden eventually. The negative attitude of the family members and questioning behavior regarding this issue pushes the female to have intense emotions such as rage, profound sorrow, resentment, responsibility, seclusion, and desperation.

Three kinds of relationships have been observed in relation to subfertility and psychological factors: (i) psychological factors resulting in subfertility, (ii) subfertility leading to psychological issues, and (iii) existence of a reciprocal relationship between the two. Depression and anxiety are persistent finding in infertile females to an extent that many women have reported about an attempt to suicide. Although infertility generates a state of depression and anxiety in a couple, psychological factors have their own influence on the reproductive abilities of both partners. Depression directly affects the HPO axis, elevates the prolactin levels, and disturbs the thyroid functions. All these three changes have their impacts on fertility.

Impact of treatment

Where couples are being challenged mentally by their subfertility, fertility treatment itself is associated with high levels of depression and anxiety. The sense of uncertainty and anxiety in females at different levels of treatment or failed trials of in vitro fertilization (IVF) and ICSI increase the depression. First-time participants have lesser anxiety and depression when compared with the women undergoing repeated attempts. The result of these treatments can bless the couple with a gift for a lifetime or can add to their disturbed mental status.

The persistent stressful condition causes increased cortisol secretion by activating corticotrophin axis. Cortisol being a stress hormone belongs to the glucocorticoid family and its release is a response to a stressful condition, which in turn effects the mechanisms like gluconeogenesis, mobilization of amino acid, and cellular immunity. The HPA axis has been recognized to bring about the changes in the reproductive system in response to stress. This psychobiological pathway reacts to stress at the central level that results the secretion of corticotropic-releasing hormone (CRH), pituitary-secreted adrenocorticotropic hormone, and consequently cortisol from the adrenals.[3] CRH-induced POMC derivatives from the pituitary regulate the hypothalamic–gonadal axis while cortisol also inhibits the axis.

Additively it also suppresses the reproductive hormones by disturbing HPO axis at the hypothalamic level, by causing the inhibition of GnRH release.[4] This suppression of GnRH involves protein–protein interaction of the DNA-bound Oct1 transcription factor.[5] Furthermore, the cortisol also plays a role in regulating normal physiological mechanisms within the ovary, primarily by changing the expression of the two isoforms of 11β-HSD. Through the follicular maturation phase, the levels of active glucocorticoids are controlled by the dehydrogenase activity of 11β-HSD, while during ovulation, the 11β-HSD surges the levels of active glucocorticoids, which induces inflammation concomitant with oocyte rupture. Furthermore, regulation of steroid production, oocyte maturation, conservation, and deterioration of the corpora lutea are also some of the functions. It is evident that an optimum level of cortisol is required for ovulation. Interestingly, cortisol also regulates the mitochondrial function by altering its activity. Thus, it is not surprising to have oxidative stress developed in the presence of cortisol.[6] Oxidative stress not only leads to mitochondrial dysfunction but also results in other systemic changes.

Stress also stimulates the release of tumor necrotic factor (TNF) and natural killer cell activity. TNF induces ovarian cell apoptosis; however, NK cells' activity has been noted to be high in unexplained cases of miscarriages and subfertility.

Authors conclude with the existence of ties between stress and fertility treatment outcomes. Poor outcome of assisted reproductive treatment (ART) such as IVF has been reported due to adverse cardiovascular activity owing to stress. Females waiting for ART have been known to have four times higher levels of depression and anxiety as compared to the women without fertility problems. The level of stress is noted to start after 6 months and accelerates after one to one and a half years of subfertility and is found highest in the group with subfertility lasting for 2–3 years. However, women experiencing subfertility for 6 years seem to get accustomed to their condition and somewhat accept their debarment.

Psychotherapy and group support sessions are practiced along with the infertility treatment plan. It reduces stress and has proved to increase the pregnancy rates, but this data is still controversial. Gentle touch like massage between the partners encourages the release of oxytocin in females and is an appreciated way of stress reduction.

Socioeconomic burden

Socially, the female is considered fortunate and high-class if she is childbearing. Despite strong financial and educational status of a female, in many societies, subfertile females are not allowed to participate in a number of family and childbearing rituals. In short, the honor of being treated equally as a fertile female is seized.[7] They are being questioned in every gathering by the fertile females and given tips for how to conceive. It becomes like a taunt or insult for the female and this creates rift initially between the couple that may lead to physical abuse and later with the family, which is usually a mental harassment. As a consequence, the female demands for a separate living, extending to affect the society financially and morally, at large.

In other cases, where the legacy or inheritance is concerned, the men are forced to marry another woman, for the sake of bearing a next of kin for extension of the family. In such a case, the infertile female either suffers the burden of another woman or is agonized by a divorce to add to the incidence of unsuccessful marriages in a said society. Conclusively, this barrenness becomes a curse for the female.

The European Society of Human Reproduction and Embryology through their Task Force in Developing Countries and Infertility is employed to recognize infertility as a magnitude public health dispute. This Task Force is actively spreading awareness of causes and impact of subfertility in Third World countries and is creating the appropriate facilities required for treatments, counseling, and other services and to outsource to the poor resource societies suffering from infecundity. This struggle becomes very laborious as it is encountered by social, financial, religious, and ethnical constraints.

Systemic effects

Emotional stress has recently been linked to oxidative stress. During stress, the body experiences some level of sympathetic activity, which might increase the respiratory oxygen intake, leading to a turnover of free radicals. Increased levels of adrenaline and reduced levels of glutathione reductase in such a scenario also aids in occurrence of oxidative stress. While some authors agree upon the vulnerability of the brain to the oxidative stress as it consumes a large percentage of oxygen as compared to its size. Once the oxygen-derived metabolites rise, they damage the cellular structures and lipid constitution of the cell membrane, including the neurons and the reproductive tissues. If not countered, OS can give rise to several diseases, inclusive of chronic and degenerative diseases, and can speed up both bodily aging and acute pathologies like trauma and stroke.

In animal model experiments, it has been evident that the glutathione reductase and glyoxalase's antioxidant activity is enhanced in anxious and depressed mice. In a very recent study conducted by Faiza et al., SIRT1 levels have been found to be reduced owing to the genetic mutation, resulting in a probable decline in the antioxidant counterbalance activity against the oxidants. This mutation affects the mitochondrial antioxidant action even in the granulosa cells and causing maturation failure of the oocytes. Increased levels of ROS along with anxiety and depression predisposes to conditions like inflammation and recurrent infections.

The hyperthyroidism, obesity, increased age, and mutations can prompt oxidative stress. The existence of free radicals is capable of causing reproductive disorders, cardiovascular, and metabolic disorders including diabetes and cancers.

Alterations in immune mechanisms secondary to stress and depression also have adverse effects on the reproductive physiology. However, studies are warranted to differentiate the direct effects of depression or anxiety on reproductive outcomes from the influence of behaviors.

Obesity and hypertension are common features of PCOs, while ROS levels are found elevated in the females with unexplained infertility.

During oxidative stress when an excess of hydroxyl radical and peroxynitrite are produced, they cause intense lipid peroxidation, thus detrimental to the cell membranes and lipoproteins. Lipid peroxidation is a rather rapidly spreading chain reaction and affects a large number of lipid constituting molecules. This destruction leads to the formation of malondialdehyde and conjugated diene compound, which are known as cytotoxic and mutagenic agents.[8]. Proteins may be affected too by undergoing conformational modifications. They may lose their functional properties as well as the enzymatic capabilities. Likewise, DNA is also prone to "stress-related lesions" in the presence of oxidative stress and 8-oxo-2′-deoxyguanosine (8-OHdG) formation is the most common consequence of pernicious DNA mutation.[9] Furthermore, oxidative stress impairs the CpG island methylation, which is a key player of the gene promoter region, causing epigenetic changes.

Counseling

Subfertility and psychological stress have a very deep relationship with great complexity. Counseling plays a crucial and supportive role in the management of subfertility. Psychological stress experienced by the couples going ART, especially IVF should be acknowledged and should be talked out to release the stress by counseling. Counseling encompasses a professional rapport between an eligible counselor and a patient, who may be a distinct, a couple, or a group of people. A formal agreement is explained and is understood by both parties. Health-care workers and researchers working in infertility clinics offer emotional care and show empathy with couples as a part of their professional role, but it is necessary to recognize this by means of counseling services within their current roles.

The HFEA Code of Practice (HFEA 2008) recognizes three distinctive types of counseling, all of which must be unmistakably discriminated from the informative conversation.

Implication counseling focuses on enabling the infertile couple/person to comprehend the consequences of artificial reproductive treatments and subsequent arrangements for themselves, their relatives including the child born consequentially, or whoever affected by the donation or treatment.

Support counseling focuses on giving emotional support to the clients at times of particular stress, for example, when there is a failure to achieve a pregnancy. This may occur at any stage before, during, and after donation or treatment.

Therapeutic counseling focuses on helping people handle the implication of subfertility and its treatment, to find possible solutions for the hardships that these might be caused, and to alter their anticipations so as to cope with the outcome of such treatment methods.

In case of genetic causes, genetic counseling is the best and efficient tool for making a better choice of cost-effective treatment for better pregnancy outcomes. A lot of options of treatment and "oocyte donation" along with "egg-sharing scheme" can be discussed.

Counseling can be helpful, but researchers have not found it to be a predictor of a positive outcome of ART. Studies suggest that couples do not take counseling very open-heartedly. Many gave feedback that they could attend such sessions if they were free of charge. Where ART is an expensive choice of treatment, counseling adds to the overheads.

References

1. Rijal B, Shrestha B, Jha B. Association of thyroid dysfunction among infertile women visiting infertility center of Om Hospital, Kathmandu, Nepal. *Nepal Med Coll J.* 2011;13(4):247–249.
2. Carroll Rocha-Frigoni NA, Leão BC, Dall'Acqua PC, Mingoti GZ. Improving the cytoplasmic maturation of bovine oocytes matured in vitro with intracellular and/or extracellular antioxidants is not associated with increased rates of embryo development. *Theriogenology.* 2016;86(8):1897–1905.
3. Dickerson SS, Kemeny ME. Acute stressors and cortisol responses: a theoretical integration and synthesis of laboratory research. *Psychol Bull.* 2004;130(3):355–391.
4. Kamel F, Kubajak CL. Modulation of gonadotropin secretion by corticosterone: interaction with gonadal steroids and mechanism of action. *Endocrinology.* 1987;121(2):561–568.
5. Dubey AK, Plant TM. A suppression of gonadotropin secretion by cortisol in castrated male rhesus monkeys (Macaca mulatta) mediated by the interruption of hypothalamic gonadotropin-releasing hormone release. *Biol Reprod.* 1985;33(2):423–431.

6. Du J, Wang Y, Hunter R, et al. Dynamic regulation of mitochondrial function by glucocorticoids. *Proc Natl Acad Sci USA*. 2009;106(9):3543–3548.

7. Unisa S. Childlessness in Andhra Pradesh, India: treatment-seeking and consequences. *Reprod Health Matters*. 1999;7:54–64.

8. Frei B. *Reactive Oxygen Species and Antioxidant Vitamins*. Linus Pauling Institute, Oregon State University; 1997. http://lpi.oregonstate.edu/f-w97/reactive.html.

9. Nishida N, Arizumi T, Takita M, et al. Reactive oxygen species induce epigenetic instability through the formation of 8-hydroxydeoxyguanosine in human. *Dig Dis*. 2013;5–6(37):459–466.

Polycystic ovary syndrome and subfertility

7

Sobia Sabir Ali[a] and Rehana Rehman[b]

[a]Department of Diabetes and Endocrinology, MTI, Lady Reading Hospital, Peshawar, Pakistan,
[b]Department of Biological & Biomedical Sciences, Aga Khan University, Karachi, Pakistan

Chapter Outline

Subfertility. https://doi.org/10.1016/B978-0-323-75945-8.00007-4

Introduction

Polycystic ovary syndrome (PCOS) is a well-appreciated heterogeneous disorder of the endocrine system. It is usually detected in women of reproductive age group who present with a cluster of clinical features ranging from androgen excess (hirsutism, alopecia, and/or acne) and ovarian dysfunction (oligo-ovulation and/or polycystic ovarian morphology (PCOM) on ultrasound).[1] More recently, obesity with its associated metabolic disorders has been recognized as one of the prominent clinical features of PCOS[2] (Table 7.1).

Definition and history of the syndrome

According to American Society for Reproductive Medicine (ASRM), PCOS is defined by "the presence of any two out of three criteria i.e. oligo and/or anovulation, excess androgen activity and/or polycystic ovarian morphology on ultrasound."[3] The antiquity of PCOS can be traced back in the words of Hippocrates, "but those women whose menstruation is less than three days or is meagre, are robust, with a healthy complexion and a masculine appearance; yet they are not concerned about bearing children nor do they become pregnant."[4] In 1935, cases of amenorrhea presented with the detailed description of the syndrome. Of these, three were obese, five were hirsute, and one obese and one thin had acne.[1] Surgical exploration confirmed the characteristic features of the ovaries, which were found to be enlarged two to four times and were full of tiny fluid-filled cysts.[5] In 1947, Kierland and his team documented skin features in females with hyperandrogenism and diabetes mellitus. Later in 1957, the eponymous "Stein–Leventhal syndrome" showed an increased concentration of androgens and luteinizing hormone (LH) in women with polycystic ovaries. In 1981, the first ultrasound appearance of polycystic ovaries was documented, and by 1985, the details of ultrasound findings such as follicle number and ovarian volume were added. The ultrasound description of the Stein–Leventhal syndrome gave the name "polycystic ovarian syndrome."[6]

Table 7.1 Heirarchy of risk factors and impact of PCOS at different age groups.

Adrenarche (age 5–20 years)	Increased secretion of DHEA, inflammatory factors, and environmental exposures
Gonadarche (adolescents)	Menstrual disorders, acne, contraception, sexual health, exercise, and activity (environmental) normal
Adulthood	Menstrual irregularities (ovarian factors), hirsutism (adrenal factors), weight gain (sedentary lifestyle), infertility (anovulatory cycles), and diet (environmental)
Pregnancy	Neuroendocrine factors, risk of miscarriage, pregnancy complications (preeclampsia, gestational diabetes), large baby, and premature delivery
Late reproductive years	Metabolic factors (diet issues, type 2 diabetes, cardiovascular disease, and longevity)

Prevalence

It is possibly the most common endocrine disorder with a prevalence of 6%–20% in women of reproductive age group.[7–9] The prevalence based on Rotterdam criteria was 11.04%, National Institute of Health was 3.39%, and Androgen Excess and Polycystic Ovary Syndrome Society was 8.03%.[10] The occurrence of infertility varies between 70% and 80% usually presenting with anovulatory issues and a higher rate of recurrent miscarriages.[2,11] In Pakistan with the increasing frequency of PCOS, the rate of fertility issues is increasing correspondingly.[12]

Pathophysiology

The multifarious pathophysiology is attributed to a range of genetic and epigenetic changes, adrenal dysfunction, hypothalamic–pituitary dysfunction, insulin resistance (IR), dyslipidemia, metabolic derangements, and environmental factors like sedentary lifestyle, atherogenic tendency, and belly fat deposition.[6,7,13–16]

Hyperinsulinemia increases androgen secretion by ovaries and/or adrenal glands due to altered steroidogenesis leading to PCOS.[9] Other theories suggest: (i) increased LH secretion, (ii) hyperinsulinemia and IR, and (iii) a defect in androgen synthesis that results in increased ovarian androgen, all contributing to phenotype comprising of metabolic, hormonal, and ovulatory dysfunctions (Fig. 7.1).

1. Hormonal impairment in PCOS
    1.1. **Disordered hypothalamic regulation** of gonadotropin secretion is proposed to be one of the causes of anovulation in females with PCOS. It could be either due to main abnormality in the firing of hypothalamic gonadotropin-releasing hormone (GnRH) neurons or due to abnormal feedback control by the ovarian steroids.[17] Furthermore, progesterone-mediated negative feedback on LH in the normal luteal phase is compromised in these females, which cannot be reversed by physiological replacement of progesterone.[17] Anovulation is reinforced by hyperinsulinemia as a result of a direct action of insulin on follicular steroidogenesis as well as gonadotropin secretion. The evidence from animal models and human subjects further supports the role of kisspeptin/neurokinin B/dynorphin neural network in dysregulation of GnRH secretion.[17]
    1.2. **Hyperandrogenism** is a feature of both ovulatory and anovulatory cycles. In PCOS, androgen comes from both ovaries and adrenals, as well as the conversion of precursors in adipose tissue and skin. Theca cells secrete more androgens due to an increase in the regulatory enzyme of androgen biosynthesis (P450c17), either due to genetic defect or due to abnormalities in proliferation and follicular atresia. Overexpression of a protein in normal theca cells has also been identified in PCOS phenotype in vitro.[18] This leads to excessive serine phosphorylation of the insulin receptor, which generates a downstream defect of insulin receptor signaling and its abnormal action on glucose metabolism.[19] The extent of severity of PCOS and phenotypic abnormalities trails the degree

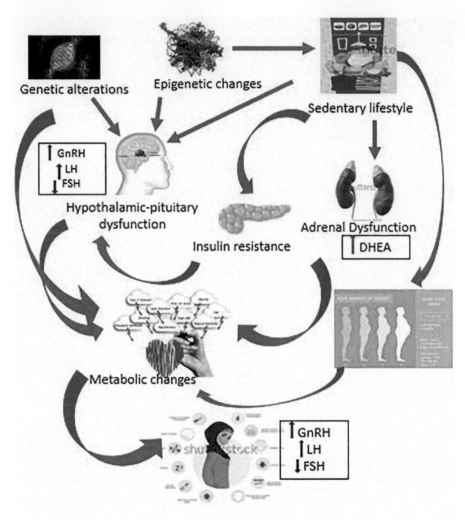

FIG. 7.1

Polycystic ovarian syndrome.

of sympathetic excitation and testosterone production.[20] Insulin also acts synergistically with LH to stimulate androgen production by theca cells.[19] Hyperandrogenism in PCOS exerts a significant negative impact on endometrial blood flow and endometrial thickness and predicts low implantation rates in in vitro fertilization (IVF).[21]

1.3. Hyperinsulinemia: IR due to postinsulin receptor deficiencies and resultant hyperinsulinemia in the ovaries disrupts feedback regulation of LH and increases androgen production contributing to anovulatory infertility.[9,19,22] Various mechanisms responsible for IR are as follows:

"Excessive serine phosphorylation of the insulin receptor subunit, mutations of the insulin receptor gene or IRS-1 (substrate of the insulin receptor, phosphorylated by its tyrosine kinase (Tyr-K) activity), depletion of intracellular adenosine, postreceptor defect of glucose transport, and impaired insulin clearance in peripheral tissues."[23] In some patients, hyperinsulinemia is contributed by a secretory pancreatic defect even in the absence of glucose intolerance or a frank type 2 diabetes mellitus (DM).[24] The growing follicle therefore is exposed to increased LH, insulin, androgen, and AMH concentrations with insufficient FSH concentrations.

1.4. **Disturbed LH–FSH ratio:** Due to increased frequency of GnRH secretion, there is an increase in 24-h secretion of LH pulse frequency and amplitude. Increased levels of LH are partly due to altered negative feedback exerted by androgens on the hypothalamic–pituitary axis.[25] Decrease in FSH due to either disturbance in hypothalamic–pituitary feedback (partial desensitization) and/or increased inhibin B production by multiple follicles has also been observed in females with PCOS.[14] Studies have demonstrated a potent inhibition of FSH-induced estrogen production in granulosa cells (GCs) by epidermal growth factor and transforming growth factor alpha 1.[5]

1.5. **Growth factors:** The deficiency of growth differentiation factor 9 has been proposed to arrest folliculogenesis before the GCs are capable of apoptosis.[19] Alterations of tumor necrosis factor α (TNF-α) in the follicular fluid have been associated with poor-quality oocytes in women undergoing assisted reproductive techniques (ARTs).

2. Ovarian dysregulation in PCOS

2.1. **Abnormal folliculogenesis and steroidogenesis:** Ovarian dysregulation occurs due to imprecise interplay of the endocrine, paracrine, and autocrine factors, leading to arrest of antral follicle development before the preovulatory stage of follicles.[19,22] Folliculogenesis in anovulatory cycles is characterized by failure of dominance, and the ovary has multiple small follicles, which are arrested but are capable of steroidogenesis. This intrinsic abnormality of folliculogenesis with altered steroidogenesis may be the root cause of anovulation in PCOS.[26] The proportion of primordial follicles is decreased with a reciprocal increase in the proportion of primary follicles.[27] The GCs of the dominant follicle acquire LH receptors, which increase LH responsiveness of GCs signals to a sequence of events that include resumption of meiosis, rupture of the ovulatory follicle, and formation of the corpus luteum. The "switch" from FSH to LH responsiveness in GCs causes an amplification of the cyclic adenosine monophosphate (cAMP) signaling pathway. Increase in intraovarian androgens induced by FSH and LH increases the chance of premature arrest of GC proliferation the same way as cAMP.[17] High serum estradiol concentrations in anovulatory cycle exert a negative feedback to suppress FSH levels.[26] The ovarian stroma in females with PCOS is more stiff and rigid, and the structural framework is not provided (Fig. 7.2).

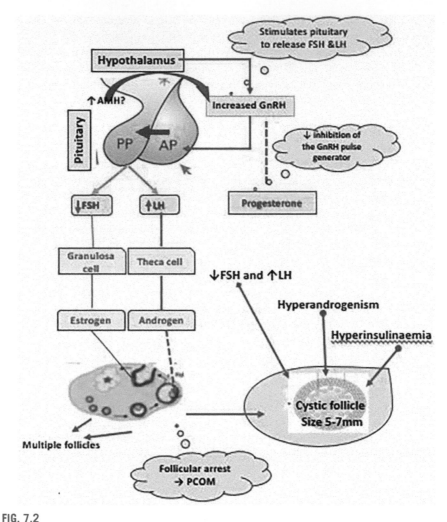

FIG. 7.2

Follicular arrest in PCOS.

2.2. Polycystic ovarian morphology (PCOM): In these women, there is increased transition from primordial to growing follicles up to an average follicular diameter of 3–5 mm with premature growth arrest, giving phenotype of enlarged ovaries with string-of-pearl morphology.[28] Ultrasound examination shows an increase in the number of follicles (2–8), hyperechogenic stromal enlargement, and multiple small follicles that are 2–8 mm in diameter, either arranged around the periphery or distributed throughout the stroma.[6] Improved understanding of the presentation of ultrasound findings in young women is needed.[29] The diagnosis of PCOS requires the presence of an ovarian volume $\geq 10\,mL$ (preferred criterion when using transducer frequencies $< 8\,mHz$) and/ or 25 follicles per ovary (criterion preferred when using transducers with frequencies $\geq 8\,mHz$).[7,30,31] In view of its potential to cause adverse psychosocial consequences, the overdiagnosis of PCOS must be prevented by strictly adhering to the diagnostic criteria for PCOM.[32]

3. Factors associated with PCOS

   3.1. PCOS and body weight: Obesity is known to intensify PCOS[33,34] and vice versa, and patients with PCOS have an increased tendency to gain weight with a fat distribution more on the upper body. However, the mechanism underlying this association is yet to be determined. Although visceral adiposity and higher BMI are positively correlated with IR, its consequential effects on other interlinked features of PCOS like menstrual disturbances and hirsutism still remain unexplained. The obesity, rather than the menstrual cycle pattern or the size of the follicular cohort, determines hyperinsulinemia, dyslipidemia, and hypertension with advancement in age.[5,6] Increase in BMI is considered to exert a negative impact on the reproductive outcome in these patients; therefore, these females are recommended to maintain BMI for improved outcomes of IVF/ICSI.[35] Dyslipidemia, IR, appearance of acanthosis nigricans, impaired lipid profiles, and glucose tolerance are more noticeable in obese PCOS as compared to lean ones.[36]

   3.2. PCOS and metabolic disorders (MetS): MetSis most frequently observed in classic NIH PCOS phenotype involving hyperandrogenism and chronic anovulation. However, women screened on the basis of Rotterdam classification having regular cycles have lesser likelihood of metabolic abnormalities.[37,38] The underlying mechanisms of IR in PCOS differ from those in other common insulin-resistant conditions like obesity and type 2 DM. Distorted secretions of adipokines like adiponectin, leptin, and resistin are supposed to cause IR, cardiovascular diseases, and metabolic disorders.[36] Women with PCOS and a combination of MetS would exhibit greater IR, higher levels of free testosterone, lower levels of sex hormone-binding globulin (SHBG), and, phenotypically, greater frequency of acanthosis nigricans.[23] Women with PCOS are at increased risk of endothelial dysfunction, altered lipid profile (increased triglycerides and low-density lipoproteins), hypertension, atherosclerosis, cardiovascular diseases like myocardial infarction, chronic obstructive pulmonary disease, autoimmune diseases, and obstetric complications.[39,40]

   3.3. PCOS and glucose disorders: PCOS is inherently related to metabolic disorders during the later course of disease. Impaired glucose tolerance or prediabetes and type 2 DM have been diagnosed in up to 40% of women with classic PCOS by the fourth decade of life, rising further with increase in age and BMI. The risk for dysglycemia was also found to be 12% in lean women with PCOS,[1] suggesting routine screening for glucose disorders. The Androgen Excess Society in 2010 issued a consensus statement on performing a 2-h post 75 g Oral Glucose Challenge in subjects of PCOS with glucose impairment.[1,2]

3.4. **PCOS and pregnancy loss:** As compared to controls, patients with PCOS exhibit an increased risk of pregnancy complications such as pregnancy-induced hypertension, preeclampsia, gestational diabetes, and premature delivery. Recurrent pregnancy loss is defined as two or more consecutive pregnancy losses before 20th week of pregnancy.[41] The prevalence of miscarriage is increased after both spontaneous and induced ovulation compromising fertility.[19] Obesity, raised serum LH levels, hyperandrogenemia, high blood glucose levels, endothelial dysfunction, and IR have been reported to be risk factors of pregnancy loss and secondary infertility.[19,42]

3.5. **PCOS and vitamin D deficiency (VDD):** The prevalence of VDD is associated with metabolic and endocrine disorders in PCOS.[34,43,44] Vitamin D (VD) is believed to affect the progression of PCOS through gene transcription and hormonal variation, influencing insulin secretion and fertility regulation.[45] VD status appears to be closely linked to IR, so much so that its supplementation is predicted to improve insulin sensitivity.[44,46,47] Replete VD status is associated with an optimal endometrial thickness and increased number of antral follicles in PCOS women during treatment cycles.[48,49]

3.6. **Hyperandrogenism:** Hirsutism is an important feature of hyperandrogenism present in approximately 70% of women with PCOS. Other features such as alopecia and acne may or may not be present. The clinical presence of hirsutism requires biochemical confirmation of hyperandrogenemia[50] by estimating serum concentration of free testosterone, determined by reliable methods only,[51] since it reflects both ovarian and metabolic disturbances.[52] A valid alternative can be the estimation of Free Androgen Index from the circulating concentrations of SHBG and total serum testosterone. Estimation of androstenedione (A4), a steroid precursor of testosterone, can be used for excess androgen levels. Hyperandrogenism leads to menstrual irregularities in the younger age group with approximately 90% chance of developing PCOS.[50,53,54] Menstrual cycles in women with PCOS tend to become more regular toward the age of menopause.[55]

3.7. **Anti-Mullerian hormone (AMH):** The utility of AMH as an indicator of screening for PCOS is still under argument because of the absence of the standardization and correct cutoff levels for different assays available for testing.[30,56] Estimation may be useful in predicting ovarian follicle counts in patients with PCOS as well as healthy women.[1,57]

Criteria for the diagnosis of PCOS

Although PCOS is often characterized by raised LH levels, fasting insulin and reversed LH–FSH ratios cannot be regarded as a diagnostic criterion. Serum testosterone levels, serum TSH, prolactin, and day 3 FSH should be done to investigate menstrual irregularities and infertility. The confirmation of diagnosis mostly relies on ruling out other causes of anovulation, including thyroid disease, 21-hydroxylase deficiency, hyperprolactinemia, Cushing syndrome, and androgen-producing neoplasms. Exclusion of other etiologies of androgen excess and/or anovulatory infertility is necessary while using any criteria for diagnosing PCOS.

1. **The Rotterdam criteria** are widely accepted and require the inclusion of two out of three features:
    1. Oligo- or anovulation,
    2. Clinical or serum indications of hyperandrogenism, and
    3. PCOM.[58,59]
2. **The NIH 2012 criteria** essentially include the same criteria as Rotterdam; however, it further classifies PCOS into four phenotypes:
    1. Phenotype A—hyperandrogenism + ovulatory dysfunction + PCOM,
    2. Phenotype B—hyperandrogenism + ovulatory dysfunction,
    3. Phenotype C—hyperandrogenism + PCOM, and
    4. Phenotype D—ovulatory dysfunction + PCOM (Table 7.2).

Table 7.2 Diagnostic criteria for PCOS.

Year	Diagnostic criteria	Diagnostic features	Number of features required for diagnosis
1990	National Institute of Health[60]	• Hyperandrogenism • Oligo- or anovulation	Two out of two
2003	Rotterdam criteria[59,61]	• Hyperandrogenism • Ovulatory dysfunction • Polycystic ovarian morphology	Two out of three
2006	AE-PCOS[7,62]	• Hyperandrogenism • Ovulatory dysfunction	Two of two
2012	NIH 2012 extension of ESHRE/ASRM 2003[50]	• Hyperandrogenism • Ovulatory dysfunction • Polycystic ovarian morphology	Two of three Identification of specific phenotype

Management of PCOS

Principles of treatment

The general principle is to individualize the treatment in accordance with the patient's need and preferences.[63] Treatment is targeted to symptoms, and in milder cases, only follow-up and observation of patient's concerns may be done over the course of years. The goals for pharmacological treatment might include improvement in features of hyperandrogenism, ovulatory dysfunction, and MetS with IR in view to address the ever-changing subjective needs, circumstances, and hopes of every patient at an individual level.[63] Preconception counseling in women with PCOS needs to be properly assured, so that the causal risk factors for reproductive failure may be detected and corrected before the commencement of medical treatment (Fig. 7.3).

Lifestyle modifications

Counseling on lifestyle modifications (LSMs) can improve menstrual cycle disorders, IR, and signs of hyperandrogenism (hirsutism and acne) with noteworthy improvements in ovarian morphology, and ovulatory cycles, mainly through decreasing plasma TNF-α, and increasing plasma interleukins (IL) IL-4 and IL-10.[64] A three-component intervention package comprising of selection of diet, exercise, and cognitive behavioral therapy is considered to improve emotional well-being of these patients.[65] It is also recommended to quit smoking and take supplemental folate.[50]

In obese females desirous of pregnancy, weight loss is the first line of therapy recommended ahead of initiating any treatment, since it has an overall effect on general

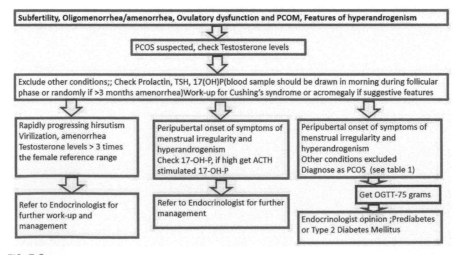

FIG. 7.3

Algorithm for diagnostic work-up of suspected PCOS.

health and prevents anovulatory cycles, pregnancy loss, complications in later days of pregnancy, e.g., preeclampsia and gestational diabetes,[50] and problems with conception like treatment failure or late response to the treatments.[66]

Management of hyperandrogenism

In women with PCOS, hirsutism is essentially treated with a variety of cosmetic techniques that may be coupled with topical and/or oral medications. The general approach includes depilatory methods like plucking, waxing, shaving, bleaching, chemical treatment, or the latest though expensive methods such as photoepilation and electrolysis.[31] The antiandrogens are the preferred drugs of choice for hirsutism, severe alopecia, and acne; retinoids have been recognized as the most effective drugs for acne.[1,31] The range of treatment depends on the severity of hirsutism and its consequential effects on fertility.[31]

Management of IR and obesity

LSM is usually recommended to prevent subsequent cardiometabolic risks with PCOS.[63] The use of different antiobesity drugs has been noted to have short-term benefits. Lately, bariatric surgery is used to treat obesity in women with MetS or its complications and PCOS. The indications for bariatric surgery are the same as that for the general population (i.e., BMI $\geq 40\,\text{kg/m}^2$ or $\geq 35\,\text{kg/m}^2$).[7] The postoperative observations have been documented to have an appreciable weight loss along with biochemical reduction in ranges of total and free serum testosterone. Furthermore, the perseverance of hirsutism and ovulatory dysfunction has been recorded in as many as 53% and 96% of women, respectively.

Management of oligo-ovulation in PCOS

The clinical picture of ovulatory dysfunction is experienced as irregularities of menstrual cycle ranging from oligomenorrhea to amenorrhca and subfertility; severity varies from patient to patient. In women with severe menstrual dysfunction, there are more chances of endometrial hyperplasia or carcinoma with subsequent infertility.[1,7]

Pharmacological treatment for ovulation induction
Clomiphene citrate

The drug of choice for ovulation induction in PCOS is clomiphene citrate (CC). The advantages are its relatively low cost, oral route of administration, fewer side effects, minimal requirement for ovarian response, monitoring, and existent evidence-based clinical data on drug safety.

The mechanism by which it acts is not completely understood, but it is agreed that it blocks the negative feedback to hypothalamo-pituitary-ovarian axis, which in turn results in amplified secretion of FSH. The predictive outcome of CC treatment is influenced by factors such as obesity, hyperandrogenemia, age, ovarian volume, and menstrual status.[50] It has been observed that standard use of 500 mg of metformin with CC results can improve live birth rate as well as cause a decline in miscarriage rate.[67]

Selection of patients

CC can be prescribed to women with "anovulatory PCOS" and "normal standard FSH" and "estradiol (E2) levels." The indicators for poorer outcome include greater age of the patient and a higher BMI. The use of exogenous gonadotropins or IVF may be considered in these patients.

> **Dose:** Initial dose is 50 mg/day for 5 days, from day 2 to 5 of the natural cycle or withdrawal bleeding after progesterone supplementation. The maximum suggested dose is 150 mg/day.[50]
>
> **Monitoring:** The ultrasonic monitoring of ovulation is not considered necessary with the use of CC.[50] The general trend of practice indicates monitoring of the first cycle to adjust the dose for successive cycles.
>
> **Efficacy:** The potential for ovulation with CC is approximately 75%–80% with a conception rate greater than 20% per cycle.
>
> **Resistance:** Phenotype A was most significantly associated with clomiphene resistance compared to other phenotypes.[68]

Alternative therapies for fertility in PCOS

> **Aromatase inhibitor:** It inhibits the production of estrogen by restraining the enzyme aromatase. A combination treatment of CC with letrozole has been proposed to be used in CC-resistant PCOS patients with improvement in ovulation and clinical pregnancy rate at a lower cost with reduced risks.[68] Letrozole has also shown promising results in intrauterine insemination (IUI).[69] The incidence of ovarian hyperstimulation syndrome (OHSS) in patients with exceptionally high AMH levels was reduced by coadministration of letrozole with GnRH antagonists.[70] Letrozole has shown better ovulation rates, monofollicular development, and higher pregnancy rates.[68,71]

Insulin-sensitizing medications

Although insulin-sensitizing medications are primarily used for the treatment of diabetes, there is ample evidence for their use in the management of women with PCOS. Insulin sensitizers include drugs such as metformin, a biguanide, and the thiazolidinediones (pioglitazone and rosiglitazone). Metformin is generally well tolerated, and the remote side effect of lactic acidosis is only seen during its use in conditions that promote tissue hypoxia-like acute illnesses or in advanced stages of chronic liver or kidney disease or congestive heart failure.

> **Use of metformin:** Metformin is a preferred treatment modality for PCOS on the basis of its ability to reduce IR, androgen levels, body weight, and menstrual irregularities.[72] Metformin has been used with calcium-VD supplements in the treatment of anovulation and oligomenorrhea in patients with PCOS.[73] In PCOS, 500 mg of metformin administered three times daily increased the frequency of spontaneous ovulation, attained menstrual regularity, and improved the ovulatory

response to clomiphene induction.[74] The more recent recommendations suggest that metformin must be prescribed in patients with underlying derangement in glucose metabolism.[1,7]

Thiazolidinediones (TZDs): These insulin-sensitizing agents are the selective agonists of peroxisome proliferation-activated receptor gamma used in the management of diabetes. Out of all TZDs, only pioglitazone is widely used in clinical practice. In a recent meta-analysis of 11 studies, improvement of menstrual cycle and ovulation in pioglitazone treatment group was better than metformin group, although pioglitazone led to higher BMI than metformin, a well-known side effect of TZDs.[75]

Myo-inositol and D-chiro-inositol supplementation has been used to restore normal ovarian functions,[3] whereas myo-inositol is an insulin-sensitizing agent that can improve the quality of embryos in women undergoing various ART procedures.[4]

A combination of insulin-sensitizing agents (myo-inositol, D-chiro-inositol, and chromium picolinate), antioxidants (N-acetylcysteine and lycopene), and vitamins (VD, biotin, and folic acid) can be prescribed in obese and nonobese females with PCOS.[76]

Gonadotropin analogs

Gonadotropin therapy in low doses (37.5–75 IU/day) is used to induce ovulation with reduced stimulation. Currently, two low-dose regimens are utilized:

(i) *Step-up regimens:* These are based on a stepwise increase in FSH administration to determine the threshold for follicular development. After 1 week, if there is no response, the dose is increased. Once the growth of the follicle is noticeable, the same dose of FSH is continued.[77]

(ii) *Step-down regimen:* The threshold of FSH is attained through a loading dose, followed by a stepwise decrease after observing the development of follicle on ultrasound.[78]

Monitoring of therapies

It is important to assess the antral follicle count by ultrasound, followed by serial ovarian ultrasound to determine the number of follicles developing in response to gonadotropin stimulation. It would be of great relevance to monitor and document all follicles 10 mm or more in size, to calculate the risk of OHSS and chances of multiple conceptions. It is of utmost importance to counsel the patient about the risks of multiple pregnancies before ovulation induction with gonadotropins.[79] The decision to cancel cycles is based on the criteria that include large number of follicles, high serum estradiol concentration, and a high number of oocytes collected.[80] Cycles are considered for cancellation when estradiol > 15,000 pmol/L or > 19 medium/large follicles at the end of stimulation and > 20 oocytes collected.[80]

Laparoscopic ovarian surgery (LOS)

Surgical approaches to induce ovulation have evolved from the historical practice of wedge resection to the modern-day slight invasive techniques, using laparoscopic ovarian diathermy or LASER. The process of doing multiple ovarian punctures by diathermy or LASER is regarded as "ovarian drilling."

Indications for LOS: Specific indications include

- Anovulatory PCOS,
- Resistance to CC,
- Patients who have persistent hypersecretion of LH, and
- Women unable to undergo intensive monitoring required for gonadotropin therapy.

Widespread ovarian diathermy is not specified to prevent hyperresponsiveness to exogenous gonadotropins. Women with duration of infertility less than 3 years respond favorably to laparoscopic ovarian drilling with a good success rate.[81]

Intrauterine insemination (IUI)

IUI may also be considered as an option. Addition of GnRH antagonist in controlled ovarian stimulation/IUI cycles resulted in a lower incidence of premature luteinization but did not improve pregnancy rates.[82] Since many women are subtle to the use of ovulation induction agents, careful monitoring is crucial to reduce the risk of OHSS and the chance of multiple pregnancies.

In vitro fertilization (IVF)

In women with PCOS and ovulatory dysfunction, IVF though is not the directly prescribed treatment. Where lifestyle intervention fails with disappointment in weight reduction, failure of antiestrogen therapy, or LOS, the need for IVF together with ovarian stimulation may be a possible mode of treatment. The main problem of induction of ovulation is a 10% chance of multiple pregnancies, exclusively after this therapy; hence, gonadotropins have to be used with caution. There has been an emphasis on utilizing IVF with single-embryo transfer, with the view to prevent the risk of multiple pregnancies. The indications for IVF in women with PCOS may include other factors: infertility due to male factor, tubal damage, severe endometriosis, and preimplantation genetic diagnosis. A GnRH antagonist cycle should always be principally used in women undergoing IVF so that a GnRH trigger can be used, following the freezing of embryos.[83]

Awareness of PCOS

Awareness regarding PCOS and related fertility is very low among females. With the very first visit of a female to a clinic presenting with menstrual irregularities, the healthcare provider should initiate steps to create awareness regarding the long-term consequences of PCOS. The following measures can be adopted as a part of routine visits to develop preventive attitudes to resist complications.[84]

- Awareness through brochures, or one-on-one counseling sessions to suggest lifestyle modifications for a better quality of life. These modifications include calorie restriction, especially low-fat, high-carbohydrate diets, regular physical activity, decreased sedentary behaviors, and behavioral strategies.
- Counseling about fertility concerns to those who want conception offering them the range of choices available.
- Regular monitoring of blood pressure, glucose tolerance, cholesterol, and triglyceride levels in those who are at risk.
- Screening for depression and anxiety as and when required.

Conclusions

On the basis of the impact of PCOS on reproductive outcomes, it is important to recognize the condition at an early reproductive age for accurate diagnosis, referral, counseling, and long-term management. Considering the condition as a multifaceted multigenic condition with strong epigenetic and environmental etiologies including food and other lifestyle aspects, it is therefore recommended to advocate lifestyle behavior modifications to all women with PCOS, irrespective of reproductive age. Its proper diagnosis and clinical management for improved fertility requires solicitation of a few clear and modest principles based on current evidence-based clinical recommendations.

References

1. Escobar-Morreale HF. Polycystic ovary syndrome: definition, aetiology, diagnosis and treatment. *Nat Rev Endocrinol.* 2018;14(5):270.
2. Lizneva D, Gavrilova-Jordan L, Walker W, Azziz R. Androgen excess: investigations and management. *Best Pract Res Clin Obstet Gynaecol.* 2016;30:1e21. https://doi.org/10.1016/j.bpobgyn.2016.05.003.
3. Hanif QA, Qamar S, Aslam P, Omar H, Mustafa N, Masood S. Association of vitamin D deficiency with polycystic ovarian syndrome. *Pak Armed Forces Med J.* 2019;69(2):241–244.
4. Azziz R, Dumesic DA, Goodarzi MO. Polycystic ovary syndrome: an ancient disorder? *Fertil Steril.* 2011;95(5):1544–1548.
5. Stein IF. Amenorrhea associated with bilateral polycystic ovaries. *Am J Obstet Gynecol.* 1935;29:181–191.
6. Minocha N. Polycystic ovarian disease or polycystic ovarian syndrome: how to identify and manage—a review. *Arch Pharm Pract.* 2020;11(2):102–106.
7. Azziz R, Carmina E, Dewailly D, et al. The Androgen Excess and PCOS Society criteria for the polycystic ovary syndrome: the complete task force report. *Fertil Steril.* 2009;91(2):456–488.
8. NIH Office of Disease Prevention. *Evidence-Based Methodology Workshop on Polycystic Ovary Syndrome*; 2012. Executive summary. Available at https://prevention.nih.gov/docs/programs/pcos/FinalReport.pdf. Accessed March, 2017; 1.

9. Witchel SF, Oberfield SE, Peña AS. Polycystic ovary syndrome: pathophysiology, presentation, and treatment with emphasis on adolescent girls. *J Endocr Soc.* 2019;3(8):1545–1573.

10. Naz MSG, Tehrani FR, Majd HA, et al. The prevalence of polycystic ovary syndrome in adolescents: A systematic review and meta-analysis. *Int J Reprod Biomed.* 2019;17(8):533.

11. Melo AS, Ferriani RA, Navarro PA. Treatment of infertility in women with polycystic ovary syndrome: approach to clinical practice. *Clinics.* 2015;70(11):765–769.

12. Baqai Z, Khanam M, Parveen S. Prevalence of PCOS in infertile patients. *Med Channel.* 2010;16(3):255–260.

13. Dennett CC, Simon J. The role of polycystic ovary syndrome in reproductive and metabolic health: overview and approaches for treatment. *Diabetes Spectr.* 2015;28(2):116–120. https://doi.org/10.2337/diaspect.28.2.116.

14. Fruzzetti F, Perini D, Lazzarini V, Parrini D, Genazzani AR. Adolescent girls with polycystic ovary syndrome showing different phenotypes have a different metabolic profile associated with increasing androgen levels. *Fertil Steril.* 2009;92(2):626–634. https://doi.org/10.1016/j.fertnstert.2008.06.004.

15. Ascaso JF, Romero P, Real JT, Lorente RI, Martínez-Valls J, Carmena R. Abdominal obesity, insulin resistance, and metabolic syndrome in a southern European population. *Eur J Intern Med.* 2003;14(2):101–106.

16. Barber T, Franks S. Adipocyte biology in polycystic ovary syndrome. *Mol Cell Endocrinol.* 2013;373(1–2):68–76.

17. Franks S, Hardy K. What causes anovulation in PCOS? *Curr Opin Endocr Metab Res.* 2020;12:59–65.

18. Rosenfield RL, Ehrmann DA. The pathogenesis of polycystic ovary syndrome (PCOS): the hypothesis of PCOS as functional ovarian hyperandrogenism revisited. *Endocr Rev.* 2016;37(5):467–520.

19. van der Spuy ZM, Dyer SJ. The pathogenesis of infertility and early pregnancy loss in polycystic ovary syndrome. *Best Pract Res Clin Obstet Gynaecol.* 2004;18(5):755–771.

20. Baig M, Rehman R, Tariq S, Fatima SS. Serum leptin levels in polycystic ovary syndrome and its relationship with metabolic and hormonal profile in Pakistani females. *Int J Endocrinol.* 2014;2014. https://doi.org/10.1155/2014/132908.

21. Lord J, Thomas R, Fox B, Acharya U, Wilkin T. The central issue? Visceral fat mass is a good marker of insulin resistance and metabolic disturbance in women with polycystic ovary syndrome. *BJOG.* 2006;113(10):1203–1209.

22. Abbott D, Barnett D, Bruns C, Dumesic D. Androgen excess fetal programming of female reproduction: a developmental aetiology for polycystic ovary syndrome? *Hum Reprod Update.* 2005;11(4):357–374. https://doi.org/10.1093/humupd/dmi013.

23. Apridonidze T, Essah PA, Iuorno MJ, Nestler JE. Prevalence and characteristics of the metabolic syndrome in women with polycystic ovary syndrome. *J Clin Endocrinol Metab.* 2005;90(4):1929–1935.

24. Dunaif A, Finegood DT. Beta-cell dysfunction independent of obesity and glucose intolerance in the polycystic ovary syndrome. *J Clin Endocrinol Metab.* 1996;81(3):942–947.

25. Jonard S, Dewailly D. The follicular excess in polycystic ovaries, due to intra-ovarian hyperandrogenism, may be the main culprit for the follicular arrest. *Hum Reprod Update.* 2004;10(2):107–117.

26. Franks S, Stark J, Hardy K. Follicle dynamics and anovulation in polycystic ovary syndrome. *Hum Reprod Update.* 2008;14(4):367–378.

27. Stubbs SA, Stark J, Dilworth SM, Franks S, Hardy K. Abnormal preantral folliculogenesis in polycystic ovaries is associated with increased granulosa cell division. *J Clin Endocrinol Metab.* 2007;92(11):4418–4426.

28. Selimoglu H, Duran C, Kiyici S, et al. The effect of vitamin D replacement therapy on insulin resistance and androgen levels in women with polycystic ovary syndrome. *J Endocrinol Invest.* 2010;33(4):234–238.

29. Rosenfield RL. The polycystic ovary morphology-polycystic ovary syndrome spectrum. *J Pediatr Adolesc Gynecol.* 2015;28(6):412–419.

30. Dewailly D, Lujan ME, Carmina E, et al. Definition and significance of polycystic ovarian morphology: a task force report from the Androgen Excess and Polycystic Ovary Syndrome Society. *Hum Reprod Update.* 2014;20(3):334–352.

31. Escobar-Morreale H, Carmina E, Dewailly D, et al. Epidemiology, diagnosis and management of hirsutism: a consensus statement by the Androgen Excess and Polycystic Ovary Syndrome Society. *Hum Reprod Update.* 2012;18(2):146–170.

32. Copp T, McCaffery K, Azizi L, Doust J, Mol BW, Jansen J. Influence of the disease label 'polycystic ovary syndrome' on intention to have an ultrasound and psychosocial outcomes: a randomised online study in young women. *Hum Reprod.* 2017;32(4):876–884.

33. Ledger WL. Non-reproductive consequences of polycystic ovary syndrome. *Curr Obstet Gynaecol.* 2003;13(6):350–354.

34. Wehr E, Trummer O, Giuliani A, Gruber H-J, Pieber TR, Obermayer-Pietsch B. Vitamin D-associated polymorphisms are related to insulin resistance and vitamin D deficiency in polycystic ovary syndrome. *Eur J Endocrinol.* 2011;164(5):741–749.

35. Rehman R, Mehmood M, Ali R, Shaharyar S, Alam F. Influence of body mass index and polycystic ovarian syndrome on ICSI/IVF treatment outcomes: a study conducted in Pakistani women. *Int J Reprod Biomed.* 2018;16(8):529.

36. Canis M, Donnez JG, Guzick DS, et al. Revised American Society for Reproductive Medicine classification of endometriosis: 1996. *Fertil Steril.* 1997;67(5):817–821.

37. Moran LJ, Misso ML, Wild RA, Norman RJ. Impaired glucose tolerance, type 2 diabetes and metabolic syndrome in polycystic ovary syndrome: a systematic review and meta-analysis. *Hum Reprod Update.* 2010;16(4):347–363.

38. Johnstone EB, Rosen MP, Neril R, et al. The polycystic ovary post-Rotterdam: a common, age-dependent finding in ovulatory women without metabolic significance. *J Clin Endocrinol Metab.* 2010;95(11):4965–4972.

39. Naz MSG, Tehrani FR, Behroozi-Lak T, Mohammadzadeh F, Badr FK, Ozgoli G. Polycystic ovary syndrome and pelvic floor dysfunction: a narrative review. *Res Rep Urol.* 2020;12:179.

40. Lee TT, Rausch ME. Polycystic ovarian syndrome: role of imaging in diagnosis. *Radiographics.* 2012;32(6):1643–1657.

41. Chakraborty P, Goswami S, Rajani S, et al. Recurrent pregnancy loss in polycystic ovary syndrome: role of hyperhomocysteinemia and insulin resistance. *PLoS One.* 2013;8(5), e64446.

42. Essah PA, Cheang KI, Nestler JE. The pathophysiology of miscarriage in women with polycystic ovary syndrome. Review and proposed hypothesis of mechanisms involved. *Hormones (Athens).* 2004;3:221–227.

43. He C, Lin Z, Robb S, Ezeamama A. Serum vitamin D levels and polycystic ovary syndrome: a systematic review and meta-analysis. *Nutrients.* 2015;7(6):4555–4577.

44. Thomson RL, Spedding S, Buckley JD. Vitamin D in the aetiology and management of polycystic ovary syndrome. *Clin Endocrinol (Oxf).* 2012;77(3):343–350.

45. Mahmoudi TJF. Genetic variation in the vitamin D receptor and polycystic ovary syndrome risk. *Fertil Steril.* 2009;92(4):1381–1383.
46. Salehpour S, Hosseini S, Nazari L, Hosseini M, Saharkhiz N. The effect of vitamin D supplementation on insulin resistance among women with polycystic ovary syndrome. *JBRA Assist Reprod.* 2019;23(3):235.
47. Trummer C, Pilz S, Schwetz V, Obermayer-Pietsch B, Lerchbaum E. Vitamin D, PCOS and androgens in men: a systematic review. *Endocr Connect.* 2018;7(3):R95–R113.
48. Asadi M, Matin N, Frootan M, Mohamadpour J, Qorbani M, Tanha FD. Vitamin D improves endometrial thickness in PCOS women who need intrauterine insemination: a randomized double-blind placebo-controlled trial. *Arch Gynecol Obstet.* 2014;289(4):865–870.
49. Arabian S, Raoofi Z. Effect of serum vitamin D level on endometrial thickness and parameters of follicle growth in infertile women undergoing induction of ovulation. *J Obstet Gynaecol.* 2018;38(6):833–835.
50. Fauser B, Tarlatzis B, Rebar R, Legro R, Balen A. Consensus on women's health aspects of polycystic ovary syndrome (PCOS): the Amsterdam ESHRE. Paper presented at: ASRM-Sponsored 3rd PCOS Consensus Workshop Group. *Fertil Steril.* 2011;97:28.
51. Rosner W, Auchus RJ, Azziz R, Sluss PM, Raff H. Utility, limitations, and pitfalls in measuring testosterone: an Endocrine Society position statement. *J Clin Endocrinol Metab.* 2007;92(2):405–413.
52. Antonio L, Pauwels S, Laurent M, et al. Free testosterone reflects metabolic as well as ovarian disturbances in subfertile oligomenorrheic women. *Int J Endocrinol.* 2018. https://doi.org/10.1155/2018/7956951.
53. Kumarapeli V, Seneviratne RA, Wijeyaratne C, Yapa R, Dodampahala S. A simple screening approach for assessing community prevalence and phenotype of polycystic ovary syndrome in a semiurban population in Sri Lanka. *Am J Epidemiol.* 2008;168(3):321–328.
54. Laven JS, Imani B, Eijkemans MJ, Fauser BC. New approach to polycystic ovary syndrome and other forms of anovulatory infertility. *Obstet Gynecol Surv.* 2002;57(11):755–767.
55. Elting MW, Korsen TJ, Schoemaker J. Obesity, rather than menstrual cycle pattern or follicle cohort size, determines hyperinsulinaemia, dyslipidaemia and hypertension in ageing women with polycystic ovary syndrome. *Clin Endocrinol (Oxf).* 2001;55(6):767–776.
56. Conway G, Dewailly D, Diamanti-Kandarakis E, et al. The polycystic ovary syndrome: a position statement from the European Society of Endocrinology. *Eur J Endocrinol.* 2014;171(4):P1–P29.
57. Christiansen SC, Eilertsen TB, Vanky E, Carlsen SM. Does AMH reflect follicle number similarly in women with and without PCOS? *PLoS One.* 2016;11(1), e0146739.
58. Gainder S, Sharma B. Update on management of polycystic ovarian syndrome for dermatologists. *Indian Dermatol Online J.* 2019;10(2):97.
59. Azziz R, Carmina E, Dewailly D, et al. Criteria for defining polycystic ovary syndrome as a predominantly hyperandrogenic syndrome: an Androgen Excess Society guideline. *J Clin Endocrinol Metab.* 2006;91(11):4237–4245.
60. Zawadzski J. Diagnostic criteria for polycystic ovary syndrome: towards a rational approach. In: *Polycystic Ovary Syndrome*; 1992:39–50.
61. Balakrishnan S, Nair M. Adolescent polycystic ovary syndrome. *Indian J Pract Pediatr.* 2019;21(1):22.
62. Rotterdam ESHRE/ASRM-Sponsored PCOS Consensus Workshop Group. Revised 2003 consensus on diagnostic criteria and long-term health risks related to polycystic ovary syndrome. *Fertil Steril.* 2004;81(1):19–25.

63. Conway G, Dewailly D, Diamanti-Kandarakis E. The polycystic ovary syndrome. A position statement from the European Society of Endocrinology. *Reprod Endocrinol.* 2015;25:32–52.

64. Abdolahian S, Tehrani FR, Amiri M, et al. Effect of lifestyle modifications on anthropometric, clinical, and biochemical parameters in adolescent girls with polycystic ovary syndrome: a systematic review and meta-analysis. *BMC Endocr Disord.* 2020;20:1–17.

65. Jiskoot G, Dietz de Loos A, Beerthuizen A, Timman R, Busschbach J, Laven J. Long-term effects of a three-component lifestyle intervention on emotional well-being in women with Polycystic Ovary Syndrome (PCOS): a secondary analysis of a randomized controlled trial. *PLos one.* 2020;15(6), e0233876.

66. Qazi II, Qazi AT, Ijaz F, Jawed S, Aftab RK, Qazi SR. Relationship of obesity with insulin resistance in polycystic ovarian syndrome. *Pak J Physiol.* 2018;14(3):46–49.

67. Heathcote G, Boothroyd C, Forbes K, Lee A, Gregor M, Luscombe G. Ovulation rate after metformin and clomiphene vs clomiphene alone in polycystic ovary syndrome (PCOS): a randomized, double-blind, placebo-controlled trial. *Fertil Reprod.* 2020;2(1):32–36.

68. Ege S, Bademkıran MH, Peker N, Tahaoğlu AE, Çaça FNH, Özçelik SM. A comparison between a combination of letrozole and clomiphene citrate versus gonadotropins for ovulation induction in infertile patients with clomiphene citrateresistant polycystic ovary syndrome—a retrospective study. *Ginekol Pol.* 2020;91(4):185–188.

69. Nguyen TT, Doan HT, Quan LH, Lam NM. Effect of letrozole for ovulation induction combined with intrauterine insemination on women with polycystic ovary syndrome. *Gynecol Endocrinol.* 2020;1–4.

70. Tshzmachyan R, Hambartsoumian E. The role of Letrozole (LE) in controlled ovarian stimulation (COS) in patients at high risk to develop ovarian hyper stimulation syndrome (OHSS). A prospective randomized controlled pilot study. *J Gynecol Obstet Hum Reprod.* 2020;49(2):101643.

71. Saeed EMA, El-Omda FA, El-Tohamy MMH. Aromatase inhibitor versus clomiphene citrate for induction of ovulation in unexplained infertility. *Al-Azhar Med J.* 2020;49(2):677–686.

72. Artani M, Iftikhar MF, Khan S. Effects of metformin on symptoms of polycystic ovarian syndrome among women of reproductive age. *Cureus.* 2018;10(8), e3203.

73. Rashidi H, Toolabi M, Najafian M, Sadrian E, Safapoor N, Nazari P. The relationship of serum 25-dihydroxy vitamin D3 concentrations with metabolic parameters in non-obese women with polycystic ovarian syndrome. *Middle East Fertil Soc J.* 2016;21(4):264–268.

74. Diamanti-Kandarakis E, Kouli C, Tsianateli T, Bergiele A. Therapeutic effects of metformin on insulin resistance and hyperandrogenism in polycystic ovary syndrome. *Eur J Endocrinol.* 1998;138(3):269–274.

75. Xu Y, Wu Y, Huang Q. Comparison of the effect between pioglitazone and metformin in treating patients with PCOS: a meta-analysis. *Arch Gynecol Obstet.* 2017;296(4):661–677.

76. Advani K, Batra M, Tajpuriya S, et al. Efficacy of combination therapy of inositols, antioxidants and vitamins in obese and non-obese women with polycystic ovary syndrome: an observational study. *J Obstet Gynaecol.* 2020;40(1):96–101.

77. Dafopoulos K, Tarlatzis BC. Hormonal treatments in the infertile women. In: *Female Reproductive Dysfunction*; 2020:247–261.

78. Della Corte L, Foreste V, Barra F, et al. Current and experimental drug therapy for the treatment of polycystic ovarian syndrome. *Expert Opin Investig Drugs.* 2020;1–12. https://doi.org/10.1080/13543784.2020.1781815.

79. Du D-F, Li M-F, Li X-L. Ovarian hyperstimulation syndrome: a clinical retrospective study on 565 inpatients. *Gynecol Endocrinol.* 2020;36(4):313–317.

80. Sood A, Mathur R. Ovarian hyperstimulation syndrome. *Obstet Gynaecol Reprod Med.* 2020;30(8):251–255. https://doi.org/10.1016/j.ogrm.2020.05.004.

81. Felemban A, Tan SL, Tulandi T. Laparoscopic treatment of polycystic ovaries with insulated needle cautery: a reappraisal. *Fertil Steril.* 2000;73(2):266–269.

82. Ozelci R, Dilbaz S, Dilbaz B, Cırık DA, Yılmaz S, Tekin OM. Gonadotropin releasing hormone antagonist use in controlled ovarian stimulation and intrauterine insemination cycles in women with polycystic ovary syndrome. *Taiwan J Obstet Gynecol.* 2019;58(2):234–238.

83. Thakre N, Homburg R. A review of IVF in PCOS patients at risk of ovarian hyperstimulation syndrome. *Expert Rev Endocrinol Metab.* 2019;14(5):315–319.

84. Jena SK, Mishra L, Naik SS, Khan S. Awareness and opinion about polycystic ovarian syndrome (PCOS) among young women: a developing country perspective. *Int J Adolesc Med Health.* 2020;1. https://doi.org/10.1515/ijamh-2018-0166 [ahead-of-print].

Endometriosis and subfertility

8

Nadeem Faiyaz Zuberi[a] and Rehana Rehman[b]

[a]Department of Obstetrics and Gynaecology, Aga Khan University Hospital, Karachi, Pakistan,
[b]Department of Biological & Biomedical Sciences, Aga Khan University, Karachi, Pakistan

Chapter outline

Introduction

The lining of a woman's uterus is made up of endometrial tissue that sheds in each menstrual cycle. In endometriosis, similar tissue develops on abnormal anatomical locations such as in the pelvis or abdominal cavity. This mislaid tissue shows a similar response to the hormonal changes of each cycle and sheds blood causing inflammation, swelling, and scarring. The discomfitures of endometriosis include dysmenorrhea, dyspareunia, chronic pelvic pain, irregular uterine bleeding, and/or subfertility

Subfertility. https://doi.org/10.1016/B978-0-323-75945-8.00008-6
© 2021 Elsevier Inc. All rights reserved.

based on the premise that the fecundity rate of women with endometriosis who have not been treated for it is lower, i.e., 2%–10%,[1] as compared to the non-subfertile couples, which ranges from 15% to 20% per month.[2]

Classifications of endometriosis

Until better classification systems are developed, a classification toolbox has been proposed,[3] which includes the revised American Society for Reproductive Medicine (rASRM) classification,[4] the Enzian classification, and the endometriosis fertility index (EFI). Both rASRM classification and Enzian classification complement one another to explain the severity and level of infiltration of endometriosis. Only EFI is strictly related to endometriosis-associated infertility (Tables 8.1 and 8.2).

Theories on pathophysiology of endometriosis

The pathologic process of endometriosis and a theory that explains this process are still poorly understood and remain controversial. Regarding the origin of endometriosis and its pathogenesis, several theories based on observations can be categorized into the implants that initiate from the uterus and those that arise from areas outside the uterus. A number of concepts and pathologic mechanisms are suggested (Fig. 8.1)[5]: implantation theory,[6] metaplasia theory,[7] induction theory,[8] epigenetic theory,[9] stem cell-based theory,[10] and perineural theory.[11]

Table 8.1 ASRM point system classification of stages of endometriosis.

Stage I (1–5 points)	• Stage I is considered "Minimal"
	• The implants are small, few in number, superficial, and shallow. These stages do not necessarily correspond to the symptoms of the diseases such as pain and discomfort levels
Stage II (6–15 points)	• Referred to as "Mild" stage
	• Implants are more in number and deeper than the superficial implants
Stage III (16–40 points)	• Called "Moderate" stage with deeper implants
	• Small endometrial cysts can be present on one or both ovaries. When the tissue attached to an ovary begins to shed blood and tissue, the clotted blood takes the form of a "Chocolate Cyst"
	• Presence of filmy adhesions from scarring of tissues
Stage IV (> 40 points)	• "Severe" stages with many deep implants
	• Large cysts on one or both ovaries
	• Many dense adhesions throughout the pelvic cavity

Based on American Society for Reproductive Medicine. Revised American Society for Reproductive Medicine classification of endometriosis: 1996. Fertil Steril. 1997;67(5):817–821. Retrieved from http://www.fertstert.org/article/S0015-0282(97)81391-X/pdf.

Table 8.2 Endometriosis classification: anatomical location and infiltration in pelvis and abdominal cavity.

Category I	• Peritoneal endometriosis is the most minimal form in which only abdominal lining is infiltrated with endometriosis tissue
Category II	• Ovarian endometriosis is located within the ovaries and carries the risk of spreading endometriosis within the pelvic cavity. In the ovary, blood gets implanted in the normal ovarian tissue to form an implant called endometrioma or "Chocolate Cyst"
Category III	• Deep infiltrating endometriosis I (DIE I) infiltrates into the pelvic cavity involving organs like the ovaries, rectum, and uterus. Adhesions refer to as "frozen pelvis"
Category IV	• Deep infiltrating endometriosis II (DIE II) spreads both within and outside the pelvic cavity and may spread as far as the heart, lungs, and the brain

Based on American Society for Reproductive Medicine. Revised American Society for Reproductive Medicine classification of endometriosis: 1996. Fertil Steril. 1997;67(5):817–821. Retrieved from http://www.fertstert.org/article/S0015-0282(97)81391-X/pdf.

Pathogenesis of endometriosis

While the debate of uterine or nonuterine origin of the disease is on, a number of factors and genetic susceptibilities have been identified to support the cause and effect mechanism of endometriosis such as endocrine-disrupting chemicals and endogenous/exogenous estrogens influencing endocrine, immune, stem/progenitor cells, epigenetic modifications[12] (Fig. 8.2).

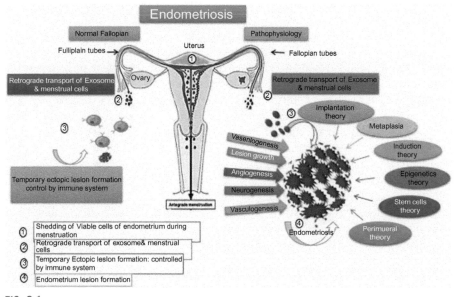

FIG. 8.1

Endometrium with respective theories.

Reproduced with permission from Azhar A, Ali R, Raja MHR, Baig R, Rehman R. Diagnosis of endometriosis in the light of prevalent theories. J Bahria Univ Med Dental Coll. 2019;9(4):316–320.

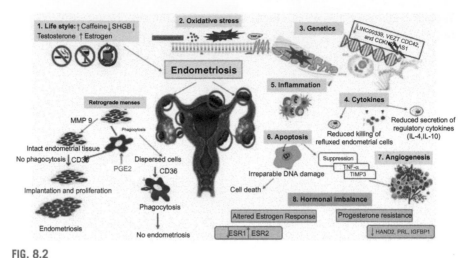

FIG. 8.2

Pathogenesis of endometriosis.

Association between endometriosis and subfertility

Association between subfertility with minimal and mild endometriosis (stage I/II) is frequently seen in cases of unexplained infertility.[13] Nevertheless, the impact of such lesions on fecundity is quite debatable. The literature suggests that although these lesions impair ovarian reserve, luteal function, and fertilization rate, the outcome is not affected in infertile females undergoing assisted reproductive technology (ART) treatment.[14] On the other hand, the association between moderate and severe endometriosis (stage III/IV) seems more plausible, because of the presence of distorted uterine tubes and ovaries leading to blockage of embryos and gametes reaching the uterine cavity. Furthermore, there is an alteration in the structural tissue of seemingly normal ovarian cortex leading to reduced ovarian reserve.[15] This could be as a result of complex interplay between various mechanisms including compromise in the vascular and nerve supply of whole ovarian complex, fibrosis changing the mechanical force and hence stimulating signaling pathways in follicular cells, and endometriotic cells themselves producing altered levels of substances, which can trigger granulosa cell activation and premature follicular development.[16] Nevertheless, as a paradox, ovarian reserve evaluated by antral follicle count is not affected following surgical management of ovarian endometrioma, while it is reduced when evaluated by serum anti-Mullerian hormone (AMH), leading to uncertainties[17] (Fig. 8.3).

The endometrial factor can itself be a confounder or has interaction between the complex interplay of endometriosis and subfertility. The eutopic endometrium in women with endometriosis is different than others. Structural and ultrastructural analysis of endometrium suggests a proliferative phase defect among women with

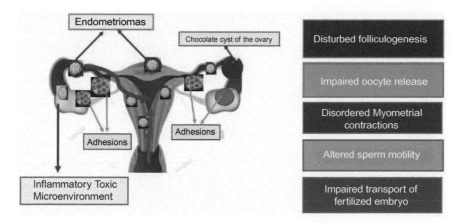

FIG. 8.3

Possible causes of reduced fertility in women with endometriosis.

endometriosis leading to low endometrial plateau thickness and a heterogeneous response to endometriosis. Endometrial nerve fibers have been documented in women with endometriosis along with their presence in the myometrium, which may play a significant role in pain generation and pelvic adhesion formation.[18,19] Increased concentrations of complement components have been reported, and dysregulation of these gene products could cause impaired implantation.[20] On the one hand, endometrial receptivity and pregnancy rates are not reduced in oocyte donation recipients affected by endometriosis, while on the other, ovarian suppression with the use of a gonadotropin-releasing hormone (GnRH) agonist or oral contraceptive before the application of an ART significantly improved implantation rates[21] leading to further uncertainties.

Issue of causality

"Endometriosis causes subfertility"—the establishment of this causal relationship requires the understanding of the type of association between these two, presence of temporal relationship, dose–response gradient, whether the association makes sense, and the effect of removal of cause.[22] Evidence from experiments in animals suggests the presence of relationship,[23] while data from experiments in humans are not available. The strength of the association in humans comes mainly from retrospective data, suggesting a greater prevalence of endometriosis in infertile females as compared to the fertile ones.[20] There is moderate comparability of groups and outcomes for endometriosis and subfertility, and there is consistent association for endometriosis vs no endometriosis in terms of increase in prevalence,[24] decrease in spontaneous conception,[25] decrease in reproductive outcome of intrauterine insemination (IUI),[26] and decrease in outcome of ART.[27,28] The temporal relationship between endometriosis and subfertility has been shown in a large cohort study in which longitudinal prospective data were collected.[29] Despite limitations of classification systems for endometriosis, a dose–response gradient cannot be disregarded as indicated in a systematic review and meta-analysis.[30] Furthermore, epidemiological and biological data also make sense as reviewed in the synthesis literature.[31,32] Lastly, the removal of endometriosis as the cause has shown that the spontaneous pregnancy rates were better after laparoscopic surgery as compared to expectant management.[33]

Evaluation process for subfertility management
Ruling out malignancy

Malignancy is not very commonly associated with endometriosis; nevertheless, it is the first thing that requires to be excluded. There remains a 0.8%–0.9% risk of occult malignancy in endometriotic cysts, while significant increased risk of low-grade serous,[34] clear cell endometrioid ovarian cancers has been documented in the literature.[35] In case, a malignant potential is identified in the mass consistent with endometrioma; oophorectomy or ovarian cystectomy can be performed along with egg or embryo freezing.

Dealing with concurrent pelvic pain

Pain is the most frequent presentation with ovarian endometrioma, while fertility desire or associated subfertility is an equally common concern among these women. For the associated pain among women also seeking subfertility treatment, cystectomy has been shown to be superior to fenestration and coagulation in terms of symptoms recurrence and need for subsequent reoperation.[36] Furthermore, pelvic pain associated with coexisting peritoneal lesions is also required to be treated along with subfertility management.[37]

Deciding the cutoff of endometrioma size for surgery

Size of ovarian endometrioma influences ovarian response in spontaneous cycles as well as in in vitro fertilization (IVF)/intracytoplasmic sperm injection (ICSI) cycles. It has been shown in a systematic review that endometrioma ≥ 3 cm is associated with lower oocyte retrieval and higher cancellation rate as compared to endometrioma < 3 cm.[27] Furthermore, implantation and clinical pregnancy rates were shown to be reduced among women with endometrioma ≥ 3 cm.[38] In a multicentric comparative study, similar progressively increasing pregnancy rates at 24 and 36 months were shown when ovarian endometrioma > 3 cm was treated with either plasma energy or cystectomy.[39] Hence, small ovarian endometrioma should not be removed prior to IVF/ICSI.[33]

Impact of ovarian cystectomy

Ovarian cystectomy has an impact on fertility, with the literature suggesting a decrease in AMH levels after surgery for up to 6–9 months.[40] This decrease is more marked in cases of bilateral as compared to unilateral endometrioma.[41] Although the decrease in ovarian reserve following ovarian cystectomy was attributed to thermal damage to ovarian parenchyma and surgical-related local inflammation, evidence is available for the impact following removal of healthy ovarian cortex during surgery.[42] A number of studies have shown that ovarian responsiveness to hyperstimulation in unoperated women with unilateral endometriomas is similar in affected as well as in the intact ovary.[43] It is important to note that bipolar diathermy is a consistent common factor affecting reduction in the serum AMH levels following ovarian endometrioma surgery.[44]

Impact of conservative management

Conservative management may itself interfere with ovarian responsiveness for controlled ovarian stimulation,[45] oocyte competence,[46] and pregnancy outcome.[47] It has also been seen that there is a progressive decline in ovarian reserve in terms of AMH levels, which is faster than that in healthy women.[48]

Treatment strategies for subfertility

The management of endometriosis in infertile women remains debated. The role of IVF has increased in recent years. Nonetheless, IVF may not be able to gratify all the damaging effects of endometriosis and can actually fail.[49]

Nonsurgical management

As medical therapies for endometriosis inhibit ovulation options, they do not provide any direct benefit to these women. Hence, therapies like progestins, combined estrogen-progestins, danazol, aromatase inhibitors, GnRH agonists, and antagonists though beneficial for endometriosis suppression are not helpful in subfertility treatments. A large systematic review of randomized control trials[30] has reported that there is no evidence to suggest that ovulation suppression is superior to placebo among subfertile women with stage I/II endometriosis who plan for conception. Medical therapy before or after surgery for endometriosis has not shown to improve fertility.[50] Nevertheless, postoperatively, it is used as a method of clearing or suppressing residual endometriosis in women in whom resection is incomplete.[1,30]

Surgical management for early-stage disease

Laparoscopic ablation of endometrial deposits in stage I/II endometriosis has been associated with a minimal yet significant improvement in live birth rates.

In Italian[50] and Canadian[51] studies, baseline untreated pregnancy rates of 22% in 52 weeks and 17% in 36 weeks, respectively, have been shown. The combined results of these two studies in a systematic review showed that there was no significant statistical heterogeneity, and the overall absolute difference is 8.6% in favor of therapy.[52]

Surgical management for advanced stage disease

Instead of cyst drainage and coagulation for stage III/IV endometriosis, laparoscopic cystectomy for endometriomas larger than 4 cm has been found to improve fertility.[53] In these women, if no other infertility factors are identified, conservative surgery with laparoscopy and if required laparotomy is likely to increase fertility.[54] This type of surgery, however, may cause a potential loss of viable ovarian cortex.[55] Women requiring repeat surgeries may be offered ART since additional surgeries can rarely increase the chances of pregnancy.[56]

Surgical management along with sclerotherapy with ethanol

The standard treatment for patients who have no symptoms or are with ovarian endometriomas >5 cm is laparoscopic stripping of cyst wall.[57] Recurrence ranges between 6% and 30% after 2 years,[58] and surgery also has a deleterious effect on ovarian reserve.[59] Ultrasound guided[60] or laparoscopic aspiration and sclerotherapy technique can be used for the management of benign-appearing ovarian cysts. Recurrence for this strategy has been reported at 0% to 62.5%[61] after 12–24 months of follow-up. The aspiration and sclerotherapy with ethanol may be followed by ovarian suppression with progesterones. If required, ovarian cystectomy at a later date may be performed with less deleterious effects on ovarian reserves.

Superovulation/IUI

In women who have had a surgical diagnosis, superovulation/IUI may be recommended. IVF may be offered as an alternate to further surgical therapy in stage I/II endometriosis.[62]

In vitro fertilization

For ART, discrepancy exists between Society for Assisted Reproductive Technology data and the results from the meta-analysis. Observational studies have shown that infertile women with endometriosis had lower pregnancy rates with IVF than those with tubal factor infertility,[28] while a later report of IVF-embryo transfer showed that the average delivery rate per retrieval for all the diagnoses was very similar to the women with endometriosis.[63]

References

1. Hughes EG, Fedorkow DM, Collins JA. A quantitative overview of controlled trials in endometriosis-associated infertility. *Fertil Steril.* 1993;59(5):963–970.
2. Chandra A, Mosher WD. The demography of infertility and the use of medical care for infertility. *Infertil Reprod Med Clin North Am.* 1994;5(2):283–296.
3. Johnson NP, Hummelshoj L, Adamson GD, et al. World Endometriosis Society consensus on the classification of endometriosis. *Hum Reprod.* 2017;32(2):315–324.
4. Canis M, Donnez JG, Guzick DS, et al. Revised American Society for Reproductive Medicine classification of endometriosis: 1996. *Fertil Steril.* 1997;67(5):817–821.
5. Azhar A, Raja MHR, Baig R, Rehman R. Diagnosis of endometriosis in the light of prevalent theories. *J Bahria Univ Med Dental Coll.* 2019;9(4):316.
6. Sampson JA. The development of the implantation theory for the origin of peritoneal endometriosis. *Am J Obstet Gynecol.* 1940;40(4):549–557.
7. Fujii S. Secondary mullerian system and endometriosis. *Am J Obstet Gynecol.* 1991;165(1):219–225.
8. Levander G, Normann P. The pathogenesis of endometriosis; an experimental study. *Acta Obstet Gynecol Scand.* 1955;34(4):366–398.
9. Koninckx PR, Barlow D, Kennedy S. Implantation versus infiltration: the Sampson versus the endometriotic disease theory. *Gynecol Obstet Invest.* 1999;47(suppl. 1):3–9. Discussion 9–10.
10. Perillo A, Bonanno G, Pierelli L, Rutella S, Scambia G, Mancuso S. Stem cells in gynecology and obstetrics. *Panminerva Med.* 2004;46(1):49–59.
11. Roth LM. Endometriosis with perineural involvement. *Am J Clin Pathol.* 1973;59(6):807–809.
12. Burney RO, Giudice LC. Pathogenesis and pathophysiology of endometriosis. *Fertil Steril.* 2012;98(3):511–519.
13. Brichant G, Audebert A, Nisolle M. Minimal and mild endometriosis: which impact on fertility? *Rev Med Liege.* 2016;71(5):236–241.
14. Kitaya K. Effect of early endometriosis on ovarian reserve and reproductive outcome. *Front Biosci (Schol Ed).* 2015;7:40–45.
15. Kitajima M, Defrère S, Dolmans M-M, et al. Endometriomas as a possible cause of reduced ovarian reserve in women with endometriosis. *Fertil Steril.* 2011;96(3):685–691.
16. Kitajima M, Dolmans M-M, Donnez O, Masuzaki H, Soares M, Donnez J. Enhanced follicular recruitment and atresia in cortex derived from ovaries with endometriomas. *Fertil Steril.* 2014;101(4):1031–1037.
17. Muzii L, Di Tucci C, Di Feliciantonio M, Marchetti C, Perniola G, Panici PB. The effect of surgery for endometrioma on ovarian reserve evaluated by antral follicle count: a systematic review and meta-analysis. *Hum Reprod.* 2014;29(10):2190–2198.
18. Tokushige N, Markham R, Russell P, Fraser IS. Nerve fibres in peritoneal endometriosis. *Hum Reprod.* 2006;21(11):3001–3007.
19. Zhang X, Yao H, Huang X, Lu B, Xu H, Zhou C. Nerve fibres in ovarian endometriotic lesions in women with ovarian endometriosis. *Hum Reprod.* 2010;25(2):392–397.
20. Matsuzaki S, Canis M, Darcha C, Pouly J-L, Mage G. HOXA-10 expression in the midsecretory endometrium of infertile patients with either endometriosis, uterine fibromas or unexplained infertility. *Hum Reprod.* 2009;24(12):3180–3187.

21. de Ziegler D, Pirtea P, Galliano D, Cicinelli E, Meldrum D. Optimal uterine anatomy and physiology necessary for normal implantation and placentation. *Fertil Steril.* 2016;105(4):844–854.

22. Tomassetti C, D'Hooghe T. Endometriosis and infertility: insights into the causal link and management strategies. *Best Pract Res Clin Obstet Gynaecol.* 2018;51:25–33.

23. D'Hooghe TM. Clinical relevance of the baboon as a model for the study of endometriosis. *Fertil Steril.* 1997;68(4):613–625.

24. D'Hooghe TM, Debrock S, Hill JA, Meuleman C. Endometriosis and subfertility: is the relationship resolved? In: *Paper presented at Seminars in Reproductive Medicine*; 2003.

25. Akande VA, Hunt LP, Cahill DJ, Jenkins JM. Differences in time to natural conception between women with unexplained infertility and infertile women with minor endometriosis. *Hum Reprod.* 2004;19(1):96–103.

26. Nuojua-Huttunen S, Tomas C, Bloigu R, Tuomivaara L, Martikainen H. Intrauterine insemination treatment in subfertility: an analysis of factors affecting outcome. *Hum Reprod.* 1999;14(3):698–703.

27. Hamdan M, Dunselman G, Li T, Cheong Y. The impact of endometrioma on IVF/ICSI outcomes: a systematic review and meta-analysis. *Hum Reprod Update.* 2015;21(6):809–825.

28. Barnhart K, Dunsmoor-Su R, Coutifaris C. Effect of endometriosis on in vitro fertilization. *Fertil Steril.* 2002;77(6):1148–1155.

29. Prescott J, Farland L, Tobias D, et al. A prospective cohort study of endometriosis and subsequent risk of infertility. *Hum Reprod.* 2016;31(7):1475–1482.

30. Hughes E, Brown J, Collins JJ, Farquhar C, Fedorkow DM, Vanderkerchove P. Ovulation suppression for endometriosis for women with subfertility. *Cochrane Database Syst Rev.* 2007;(3). CD000155.

31. De Ziegler D, Borghese B, Chapron C. Endometriosis and infertility: pathophysiology and management. *Lancet.* 2010;376(9742):730–738.

32. Tanbo T, Fedorcsak P. Endometriosis-associated infertility: aspects of pathophysiological mechanisms and treatment options. *Acta Obstet Gynecol Scand.* 2017;96(6):659–667.

33. Dunselman G, Vermeulen N, Becker C, et al. ESHRE guideline: management of women with endometriosis. *Hum Reprod.* 2014;29(3):400–412.

34. Mostoufizadeh M, Scully RE. Malignant tumors arising in endometriosis. *Clin Obstet Gynecol.* 1980;23(3):951–963.

35. Pearce CL, Templeman C, Rossing MA, et al. Association between endometriosis and risk of histological subtypes of ovarian cancer: a pooled analysis of case–control studies. *Lancet Oncol.* 2012;13(4):385–394.

36. Alborzi S, Momtahan M, Parsanezhad ME, Dehbashi S, Zolghadri J, Alborzi S. A prospective, randomized study comparing laparoscopic ovarian cystectomy versus fenestration and coagulation in patients with endometriomas. *Fertil Steril.* 2004;82(6):1633–1637.

37. Khan KN, Kitajima M, Fujishita A, et al. Pelvic pain in women with ovarian endometrioma is mostly associated with coexisting peritoneal lesions. *Hum Reprod.* 2013;28(1):109–118.

38. Coccia ME, Rizzello F, Barone S, et al. Is there a critical endometrioma size associated with reduced ovarian responsiveness in assisted reproduction techniques? *Reprod Biomed Online.* 2014;29(2):259–266.

39. Mircea O, Puscasiu L, Resch B, et al. Fertility outcomes after ablation using plasma energy versus cystectomy in infertile women with ovarian endometrioma: a multicentric comparative study. *J Minim Invasive Gynecol.* 2016;23(7):1138–1145.

40. Celik HG, Dogan E, Okyay E, et al. Effect of laparoscopic excision of endometriomas on ovarian reserve: serial changes in the serum antimüllerian hormone levels. *Fertil Steril.* 2012;97(6):1472–1478.
41. Alborzi S, Keramati P, Younesi M, Samsami A, Dadras N. The impact of laparoscopic cystectomy on ovarian reserve in patients with unilateral and bilateral endometriomas. *Fertil Steril.* 2014;101(2):427–434.
42. Romualdi D, Zannoni GF, Lanzone A, et al. Follicular loss in endoscopic surgery for ovarian endometriosis: quantitative and qualitative observations. *Fertil Steril.* 2011;96(2):374–378.
43. Benaglia L, Pasin R, Somigliana E, Vercellini P, Ragni G, Fedele L. Unoperated ovarian endometriomas and responsiveness to hyperstimulation. *Hum Reprod.* 2011;26(6):1356–1361.
44. Somigliana E, Berlanda N, Benaglia L, Viganò P, Vercellini P, Fedele L. Surgical excision of endometriomas and ovarian reserve: a systematic review on serum antimüllerian hormone level modifications. *Fertil Steril.* 2012;98(6):1531–1538.
45. Somigliana E, Benaglia L, Paffoni A, Busnelli A, Vigano P, Vercellini P. Risks of conservative management in women with ovarian endometriomas undergoing IVF. *Hum Reprod Update.* 2015;21(4):486–499.
46. Sanchez AM, Vanni VS, Bartiromo L, et al. Is the oocyte quality affected by endometriosis? A review of the literature. *J Ovarian Res.* 2017;10(1):1–11.
47. Fernando S, Breheny S, Jaques AM, Halliday JL, Baker G, Healy D. Preterm birth, ovarian endometriomata, and assisted reproduction technologies. *Fertil Steril.* 2009;91(2):325–330.
48. Kasapoglu I, Ata B, Uyaniklar O, et al. Endometrioma-related reduction in ovarian reserve (ERROR): a prospective longitudinal study. *Fertil Steril.* 2018;110(1):122–127.
49. Kistner RW. Management of endometriosis in the infertile patient. *Fertil Steril.* 1975;26(12):1151.
50. Parazzini F, Cipriani S, Bravi F, et al. A metaanalysis on alcohol consumption and risk of endometriosis. *Am J Obstet Gynecol.* 2013;209(2). 106.e101–110.
51. Marcoux S, Maheux R, Berube S. Laparoscopic surgery in infertile women with minimal or mild endometriosis. Canadian Collaborative Group on Endometriosis. *N Engl J Med.* 1997;337(4):217–222.
52. Crosignani PG, Vercellini P, Biffignandi F, Costantini W, Cortesi I, Imparato E. Laparoscopy versus laparotomy in conservative surgical treatment for severe endometriosis. *Fertil Steril.* 1996;66(5):706–711.
53. Chapron C, Vercellini P, Barakat H, Vieira M, Dubuisson J-B. Management of ovarian endometriomas. *Hum Reprod Update.* 2002;8(6):591–597.
54. Schenken R. Modern concepts of endometriosis. Classification and its consequences for therapy. *J Reprod Med.* 1998;43(suppl. 3):269–275.
55. Donnez J, Nisolle M, Gillet N, Smets M, Bassil S, Casanas-Roux F. Large ovarian endometriomas. *Hum Reprod.* 1996;11(3):641–645.
56. Pagidas K, Falcone T, Hemmings R, Miron P. Comparison of reoperation for moderate (stage III) and severe (stage IV) endometriosis-related infertility with in vitro fertilization-embryo transfer. *Fertil Steril.* 1996;65(4):791–795.
57. Deckers P, Ribeiro SC, Simões RDS, Miyahara CBDF, Baracat EC. Systematic review and meta-analysis of the effect of bipolar electrocoagulation during laparoscopic ovarian endometrioma stripping on ovarian reserve. *Int J Gynecol Obstet.* 2018;140:11–17.

58. Cranney R, Condous G, Reid S. An update on the diagnosis, surgical management, and fertility outcomes for women with endometrioma. *Acta Obstet Gynecol Scand.* 2017;96:633–643.

59. Raffi F, Metwally M, Amer S. The impact of excision of ovarian endometrioma on ovarian reserve: a systematic review and meta-analysis. *J Clin Endocrinol Metab.* 2012;97:3146–3154.

60. Garcia-Tejedor A, Martinez-Garcia JM, Candas B, et al. Ethanol sclerotherapy versus laparoscopic surgery for endometrioma treatment: a prospective, multicenter, cohort pilot study. *J Minim Invasive Gynecol.* 2020;27(5):1133–1140. https://doi.org/10.1016/j.jmig.2019.08.036.

61. Cohen A, Almog B, Tulandi T. Sclerotherapy in the management of ovarian endometrioma: systematic review and meta-analysis. *Fertil Steril.* 2017;108:117–124.e5.

62. Kemmann E, Ghazi D, Corsan G, Bohrer M. Does ovulation stimulation improve fertility in women with minimal/mild endometriosis after laser laparoscopy? *Int J Fertil Menopausal Stud.* 1993;38(1):16.

63. The Practice Committee of the American Society for Reproductive Medicine. Endometriosis and infertility: a committee opinion. *Fertil Steril.* 2012;98(3):591–598.

Thyroid imbalance and subfertility

Aisha Sheikh

Lecturer and Consultant Endocrinologist, The Aga Khan University Hospital, Karachi, Pakistan;
Medicell Institute of Diabetes, Endocrinology and Metabolism (MIDEM),
Karachi, Pakistan; Registered Tutor for Diploma in Diabetes and Endocrinology,
University of South Wales, Cardiff, United Kingdom

Chapter outline

Introduction

An optimal level of thyroid hormones is needed for reproductive health. This has been proved clearly in women who have a higher chance of having "autoimmune thyroid diseases (Hashimoto's thyroiditis and Graves' disease)" compared to men. Both overt and subclinical thyroid disease and thyroid autoimmunity (TAI) have

Subfertility. https://doi.org/10.1016/B978-0-323-75945-8.00009-8

Table 9.1 Diagnosis of thyroid dysfunction.

	TSH (0.4–4.2 mIU/L)	FT4 (0.89–1.76 ng/dL)
Euthyroid	Normal	Normal
Subclinical hypothyroidism	High	Normal
Overt hypothyroidism	High	Low
Subclinical hyperthyroidism	Low	Normal
Overt hyperthyroidism	Low	High

been shown to be associated with infertility. Thyroid dysfunction can adversely affect follicular development, spermatogenesis, fertilization rates, embryo quality, and live birth rates. The evidence of this association is clearer with hypothyroidism than hyperthyroidism. Overt hypothyroidism leads to menstrual cycle irregularity and ovulatory dysfunction. Through the negative feedback on hypothalamic–pituitary axis, it leads to hyperprolactinemia and ovulatory dysfunction resulting from interference with pulsatile release of GnRH. Thyroid dysfunction causes alteration in sex steroids and sex hormone-binding globulin (SHBG) levels; hyperthyroidism and hypothyroidism affect SHBG levels and thus can impact reproduction.

The classification of thyroid dysfunction is given in Table 9.1.

Thyroid imbalance and female subfertility
Association of thyroid dysfunction with menstrual irregularity

Both "overt hypothyroidism" and "overt hyperthyroidism" can entail menstrual irregularity like polymenorrhea, oligomenorrhea, and menorrhagia. As many as 22% of hyperthyroid women can have menstrual irregularity in comparison with 8% of euthyroid controls.[1] Infertile women with menstrual irregularities were prone to have abnormal thyroid function.[2] Among infertile women, 67% had menstrual irregularity, while only 29% fertile women had menstrual disorder.[3] In another study including 171 women with TSH concentrations >15 mU/L, menstrual irregularity was reported in 68% while only 12% women had menstrual irregularities among euthyroid controls.[4]

Association of thyroid dysfunction with subfertility

Thyroid dysfunction is frequently found in infertile women in contrast to fertile women. Infertile women had lesser chances to be euthyroid in comparison with fertile women in a study which reported that 62.6% of infertile women were euthyroid compared to 82.6% of fertile women.[3] In a study on women of reproductive age, the frequency of infertility was 52.3% and 47% in women with Graves' disease and Hashimoto's thyroiditis, respectively.[5] However, there are contradictory data as well that reported similar prevalence of subclinical or overt hyperthyroidism in both infertile and fertile women.[6] A retrospective study on 200 subfertile women aged 17–40 years revealed that 14% of women had preexisting hypothyroidism, 14.5% had recently discovered hypothyroidism, while 21% had subclinical hypothyroidism (SCH).[7]

Hypothyroidism was significantly associated with higher LH (8.5 IU/L vs 6.8 IU/L) and infertility related to anovulation (47.8% vs 27%) in women with TSH above or below 4.2 mIU/L, respectively.[77] Thus, it provides an insight into altered gonadotropin levels with hypothyroidism.

Association of SCH with subfertility

Many studies have tried to answer this question, but the results are inconsistent. A cross-sectional study found a prevalence of SCH in 2.3% of 704 infertile women, but this prevalence was comparable to background general population.[8] Similar results were reported by another prospective study in which infertile women did not have increased prevalence of SCH.[6] Nevertheless, many studies have shown increased rates of SCH in subfertile women. Higher frequency of SCH (13.9%) was found in infertile women in contrast to 3.9% in fertile women in a retrospective study.[9] Among 454 women presenting for subfertility, TSH >4.5 mIU/L was found in 24%.[10] Women with ovulatory disorders and "unexplained (UE) infertility" had the highest level of TSH, while it was lower among those women with either tubal disorders or infertility due to male factor.[11] Even euthyroid women with UE infertility had higher TSH values within the specified normal range. {TSH (mIU/L): UE infertility—1.95 vs male factor infertility—1.66; P—0.003}.[11] In addition, women with UE infertility had double the chance of having a TSH of ≥ 2.5 mIU/L in comparison with controls with male factor infertility.[12]

Association of TAI and subfertility in women

TAI identified by the existence of thyroid peroxidase antibodies (TPOAbs) or thyroglobulin antibodies (TgAbs) is frequently stated in subfertile women. Specifically, TPOAb has been related to lower fertilization rates and unstable embryogenesis.[13]

TPOAb was likely to be positive in euthyroid women having female factor infertility in comparison with fertile, age-matched euthyroid women.[6] In women with polycystic ovarian syndrome (PCOS), the frequency of TAI may be higher in comparison with controls.[14] In subfertile women with PCOS, the existence of TAI has been correlated with a lower probability of maturing ovarian follicles with the use of clomiphene citrate for ovulation induction.[15] However, other studies have failed to prove such associations. Among infertile women with PCOS, a study conducted on 436 women undergoing 530 antral follicular count (AFC) measurements, no correlation was found with regard to thyroid function or TPOAb positivity with AFC.[16] Conversely, the same study reported that lower free T3 and TPOAb positivity were coupled with a lower AFC in females with diminished ovarian reserve (DOR) or UE infertility.[16]

Consequences of "assisted reproductive technology (ART)" in women with SCH

There are inconsistent data on adverse outcomes of ART in women with SCH. Most of the evidence shows that rates of success of in vitro fertilization (IVF) for women with serum TSH <2.5 mU/L and those with TSH between 2.5 and 5 mU/L are not very different.

SCH is accompanied by DOR in women during later reproductive age. Out of 2568 women seeking infertility treatment who were more than 35 years old, SCH was considerably related to follicular-stimulating hormone (FSH), anti-Mullerian hormone concentrations, and AFC.[17]

In a prospective study of female cohort with baseline serum TSH within the range of 0.4–4.99 mU/L who went through intrauterine insemination (IUI), no association was found with variables of IUI, rates of pregnancy, and live birth in each cycle.[18] Multiple studies investigated the effect of TSH ≤ 2.5 mIU/L vs TSH > 2.5 or < 4.5 mIU/L on outcomes of ART, i.e., rates of pregnancy, miscarriages, or live births with no significant difference reported.[19,20] Similarly, aggregate of rates of pregnancy and miscarriages was comparable between women with TSH < 2.5 and 2.5–3.5 mIU/L and presence of TAI.[21] In contrast, a retrospective study of IVF on 164 women reported higher clinical pregnancy rates in women with TSH ≤ 2.5 (22%) vs those with TSH > 2.5 mU/L (9%).[22] Other researchers have looked at the difference in embryo quality during IVF cycle in women with serum TSH 0.45–2.5 mU/L vs 2.5–4.5 mU/L and observed no significant change in embryo quality, implantation, pregnancy loss, or live birth rates.[23,24] Thus, the existing evidence suggests that SCH may or may not impact outcomes of ART but at the same time highlights the fact that this impact can worsen as TSH continues to rise. Based on these data, treatment of SCH can be offered to infertile women undergoing ART for levels of > 2.5 mU/L, keeping in mind that low-dose thyroid hormone replacement is generally safe. Nevertheless, it should be noted that high-quality data verification is not available in favor of this recommendation.

Effect of treatment of SCH on ART results

Different studies have shown varying results in infertile women having SCH who received treatment. Similarly, there have been inconsistent results in women with SCH with or without TAI. However, there is general understanding based on existing scientific evidence that the treatment of substantial elevation of TSH (though still categorized as SCH) may benefit the ART outcome. Sixty-four women having SCH (TSH > 4.5 mU/L with normal FT4) undergoing IVF were randomized to levothyroxine (LT4) treatment 50 μg/day commenced during controlled ovarian hyperstimulation (COH) vs placebo. The LT4 was titrated in the treated women to attain TSH < 2.5 mU/L, and this level was maintained during pregnancy in women who became pregnant. Women treated with LT4 had greater proportions of achieving pregnancy, lesser chances of miscarriage, and superior rates of delivery.[25] Similar outcomes were observed in another randomized trial.[26] However, other studies did not show improved outcomes with LT4 treatment. A prospective study on 270 women who experienced initial IVF cycle while they were treated for SCH did not observe difference in rate of pregnancy, miscarriage, and live birth in women with basal TSH level between 0.2 and 2.5 mIU/L in comparison with those with baseline TSH level between 2.5 and 4.2 mIU/L.[27]

A recent meta-analysis of four RCTs including 787 women with TAI and SCH undergoing IVF/intracytoplasmic sperm injection (ICSI) did not find an appreciable interrelation of LT4 treatment with the clinical pregnancy rate, live birth rate, or preterm birth rate. However, women getting LT4 treatment had a suggestively lower miscarriage rate in comparison with those on placebo/no treatment (RR=0.51, 95% CI 0.31–0.82).[28] A meta-analyses of 13 studies comprising of 7970 women showed that in women having SCH; LT4 treatment lowered the chances of miscarriage in pregnancies attained by ART but not in spontaneously conceived pregnancies.[29] Cochrane database of systematic reviews included four RCTs with 850 women undergoing IVF/ICSI who were either having SCH or were euthyroid with positive TAI. Women who were already on LT4 were excluded. Women were assigned LT4 or placebo/no treatment in these RCTs. The analysis implied that women having SCH with either positive or negative TPOAb who are using LT4 had a 27% and 100% chance of live birth compared to 25% probability of a live birth in the groups receiving placebo/no treatment.[30] This was based on RCT from Kim et al. that stated that LT4 replacement in women with SCH with positive or negative TPOAb may help in improving live birth rates.[26] Due to low-quality evidence, the review did not draw a conclusion.[30]

Outcomes of ART in treated hypothyroid women as compared to healthy controls

Studies have looked at the impact of ART in women with treated hypothyroidism. A study included 240 women with age less than 37 years who went through first IVF cycles; compared to euthyroid women, inferior pregnancy rates were reported in 21 hypothyroid women well controlled on LT4 replacement.[31] Similarly, another study on women undertaking IVF/ICSI that included 137 hypothyroid women on LT4 treatment and 274 euthyroid controls did not find significant association of optimally treated hypothyroidism with lesser rates of pregnancy and live births.[32] In a countrywide study of all women who received ART in Denmark from 1994 till 2017, the chances of a pregnancy and a live birth after embryo transfer were studied. Those with thyroid imbalance were divided into two categories: hypothyroid/hyperthyroid disorders. In women with hypothyroidism, the adjusted odds ratio (aOR) was 1.03 (95% CI 0.94–1.12) for biochemical/clinical pregnancy or live birth.[33]

Consequences of ART in euthyroid women with TAI

Research on question of ART results in euthyroid women with TAI is heterogeneous and has included women with varying causes of subfertility. Only a few studies were limited to euthyroid women. In addition, there was heterogeneity in terms of ART/IVF protocols used in these studies. "Idiopathic DOR" was related to more frequent occurrence of positive TPOAb instead of thyroid imbalance or positive TgAb.[34] A meta-analysis concluded that pregnancy rates subsequent to IVF do not vary by presence or absence of TAI; however, there is advanced possibility of pregnancy loss in women with TAI.[35] No variances in pregnancy, pregnancy loss, or live birth rates in women with or without TAI undergoing IVF with ICSI were reported in few retrospective studies.[36–38] A study on euthyroid women undergoing IUI did not show any substantial variation among TPOAb positive and negative groups with regard to live birth, pregnancy, or miscarriage rate. Comparison of euthyroid women in subgroups with TSH ≥ 2.5 mIU/L vs TSH < 2.5 mIU/L failed to show any noteworthy differences in the outcomes.[39] Similar results were shown by different researchers.[40] In euthyroid women with UE infertility who do not have TAI, a preconception TSH between 0.5 and 4.5 mIU/L does not have a noteworthy impact on results of IUI.[41] In contrast, a retrospective study on women with or without TAI undergoing IVF reported that "fertilization," "implantation," and "pregnancy rates" were inferior in 90 women with TAI vs 676 women without TAI, but the details of thyroid status were not stated in each group.[42]

Correlation of follicular fluid TAI and TSH with serum TAI and TSH in women undergoing ART

Researchers examined the effect of follicular fluid TAI and thyroid function test in euthyroid TAI-positive ($n = 26$) vs euthyroid TAI-negative ($n = 26$) women undergoing ART. Among the two groups, no substantial differences were noticed between the TSH and FT4 measured in follicular fluid.[43] Considerable relationship was observed between the levels of serum thyroid and follicular fluid thyroid antibodies.[43] Pregnancy rates differed per embryo transfer cycle between TAI-positive women (34.8%) and TAI-negative women (66.7%). A further multivariate analysis indicated that TAI-positive women had reduced chances to attain pregnancy.[43] This led to the conclusion that in TAI-positive women, higher levels of thyroid autoantibodies in follicular fluid are intensely interrelated with the serum levels and may have an adverse influence on embryo development in postimplantation period.[43] In women with TAI, the follicular fluid has detectable thyroid antibodies at levels which correlate with that in the woman's serum.[44] Follicular fluid thyroid hormone levels correlate strongly with maternal serum thyroid hormone levels on the day of human chorionic gonadotropin (hCG) administration, and thyroid hormones on the hCG day may impact the ART outcome.[45] However, the data on whether thyroid antibodies can affect the fertilization potential of the maturing follicles are still lacking.

ART outcome of euthyroid women with TAI on treatment

There is a lot of controversy surrounding this question. Few studies have used prednisolone 5 mg compared to placebo in euthyroid women with TAI, and other studies have used low-dose thyroid hormones compared to placebo in randomized controlled trials. The outcomes were heterogeneous. A trial including 60 euthyroid women (TSH < 2.5 mU/L) with TAI going through IVF were given prednisolone 5 mg/day commencing from the day of ovum pickup, which was continued during the first trimester.[46] Better rates of pregnancy and live birth were observed in the women who received treatment.[46] Additional clinical trial with 48 infertile women with positive TPOAb was given prednisone vs placebo for 1 month prior to IUI.[47] The rate of pregnancy was superior (33.3%) in women who received treatment as compared to almost 8% in the placebo group.[47] There was no noteworthy difference in rates of pregnancy loss between the two groups.[47] Despite these small trials showing positive results, we are still unaware of positive recommendations for corticosteroid use in early pregnancy.[48] The "American Thyroid Association" endorses against the use of corticosteroids in euthyroid women with TAI going through ART.[49]

The use of low-dose thyroid hormones in doses of 25–50 µg daily compared with placebo in women with TAI undergoing ART has mixed results. Two studies on the use of LT4 in euthyroid women with TAI undergoing ART did not improve outcomes.[50,51] An RCT from China on 600 TPOAb-positive euthyroid women randomized to receive LT4 treatment vs no treatment; the authors did not observe a reduction in miscarriage rates or increase in live birth in either group.[52] The TABLET trial randomized 952 euthyroid women with positive TPOAb into LT4 50 µg vs placebo. The use of LT4 failed to exhibit a superior rate of live births as compared to placebo.[53] Cochrane database of systematic reviews included four RCTs with 850 women undergoing IVF/ICSI who were either having SCH or were euthyroid with positive thyroid antibodies.[30] Women who were already on LT4 were excluded. Women were assigned LT4 or placebo/no treatment in these RCTs. The evidence suggested that euthyroid women with TAI are likely to exhibit 31% probability of a live birth with placebo/no treatment and that the probability of a live birth in women receiving LT4 is likely to vary from 26% to 40%.[30] This review could not draw a conclusion due to low-quality evidence.[30]

Outcome of ART with hyperthyroidism

Little evidence is available on outcome of ART with hyperthyroidism. From Denmark, a countrywide study of women receiving ART showed that the likelihood of a biochemical pregnancy was significantly reduced (aOR=0.80, 95% CI 0.69–0.93) in women with hyperthyroidism. Thus, there was a reduced probability of a live birth per embryo transfer in hyperthyroid vs euthyroid women.[33]

Effect of COH on thyroid status

During IVF/ICSI protocols, the woman undergoes COH by the administration of "gonadotropins," "gonadotropin-releasing hormone analogs (GnRH-a)," or "gonadotropin-releasing hormone antagonists" in combination with gonadotropins. Maturation of follicles is tracked by ultrasound, and when the predominant follicles attain a sufficient size, then hCG is administered to induce ovulation. COH results in a rapid rise of serum estradiol to increased levels (4000–6000 ng/L), and these levels are similar to those observed in the third trimester of pregnancy.[54] Since estradiol increases thyroxine-binding globulin, these hormonal influences may modify thyroid function resulting in reduced FT4 levels and subsequent TSH elevation through feedback mechanisms. Additionally, hCG has structural homology to TSH and its administration can directly act on TSH receptors located on the thyroid gland albeit having a weak thyrotropin activity. This causes increased thyroid hormone levels and drop in TSH through feedback mechanism. Studies have shown inconsistent effects of COH on serum thyroid hormones. Few studies have reported increase in TSH or FT4 levels, while other studies have reported either a reduction in TSH or even no change during COH.[55–57] Elevations in serum levels of both TSH and FT4 were reported during COH that reached the maximum concentration 1 week after hCG administration.[58] As many as 44% of the women with baseline TSH below 2.5 mIU/L noticed TSH increasing to > 2.5 mIU/L.[58] This increase in serum TSH occurs in correspondence to rising estradiol levels during COH but is reported to be more marked in women with positive TPOAb.[59]

Another study investigated the impact of long-acting GnRH-a on thyroid status in 207 euthyroid women undergoing IVF/ICSI. TSH was checked at six distinct points during stimulation. 57.7% of women with baseline TSH between 0.35 and 2.5 mIU/L showed an increase in TSH after COH: As many as 2.2% had a simultaneous rise in TPOAb, 2.9% were diagnosed as SCH, and the remaining 42.3% had reduced TSH with a single woman discovered with subclinical hyperthyroidism. 74.3% of women with basal TSH of 2.5–4.5 mIU/L showed increasing trend in TSH after COH with 22.9% diagnosed as SCH and 25.7% had decreased TSH, out of whom one had a diagnosis of subclinical hyperthyroidism. Women with baseline TSH < 2.5 mIU/L had significantly greater clinical pregnancy rate than those with TSH > 2.5 mIU/L.[60] In a recent meta-analysis of 12 studies comprising of more than 7000 euthyroid women undertaking IVF/ICSI, a high TSH level > 2.5 mIU/L did not influence clinical pregnancy rate or miscarriage rate.[61] The available evidence suggests that the therapeutic regimen used for COH induces a deterioration of thyroid function and increased risk of untimely elevation of TSH during fertilization in patients who are suffering from TAI. Experts agree that a woman with TAI should have a TSH value < 2.5 mIU/L before undergoing COH and the TSH should be strictly monitored to start or increase LT4 treatment, when necessary.[62]

Studies have shown that the impact of COH on TSH is more marked in women with hypothyroidism on adequate LT4 replacement.[63] More marked TSH elevation at the time of egg retrieval is reported in hypothyroid women compared to their euthyroid counterparts.[58] In one study on hypothyroid women, basal TSH of 1.7 ± 0.7 mIU/L increased to 2.9 ± 1.3 mIU/L on the day of hCG administration and subsequently rose to 3.2 ± 1.7 mIU/L on day 16 after hCG administration.[64]

Due to these changes in TSH during COH, experts recommend against measuring TSH during COH as the levels will be difficult to interpret.[49] If needed, TSH should be measured either before COH or 1–2 weeks after COH. If TSH elevation (> 2.5 mIU/L) persists after COH and the woman is pregnant, she should receive LT4, and if pregnancy is not achieved, her TSH should be monitored within few weeks to confirm that the level has returned to baseline.[49]

Table 9.2 summarizes the management of thyroid dysfunction in women seeking subfertility management.

Table 9.2 Treatment of Thyroid dysfunction.

Check TSH in all women seeking subfertility management		
Involve endocrinologist for expert care of women with thyroid dysfunction and subfertility		
Clinical condition	**Treatment**	**Monitoring**
Euthyroid women with positive thyroid autoimmunity	No treatment	Monitor TSH every 6–12 weeks during infertility treatment with the aim to start levothyroxine (LT4) if TSH goes > 4.2 mIU/L Consider LT4 treatment to keep TSH < 2.5 mIU/L in women undergoing COH
Subclinical hypothyroidism	Treat with levothyroxine 1–1.2 μg/kg/day	Monitor TSH every 6 weeks, and adjust LT4 dose with the aim to keep TSH < 2.5 mIU/L before infertility treatment/ART/preconception
Overt hypothyroidism	Treat with levothyroxine 1.6 μg/kg/day	Monitor TSH every 6 weeks, and adjust LT4 dose with the aim to keep TSH < 2.5 mIU/L before infertility treatment/preconception
Subclinical hyperthyroidism	No treatment	Check TSH receptor antibodies Monitor TSH/FT4 every 6–12 weeks with the aim to start antithyroid drugs (ATDs) if the woman develops overt hyperthyroidism
Overt hyperthyroidism	Treat with ATDs/surgery/radioactive iodine (RAI) in consultation with endocrinologist	Monitor TSH/FT4 every 6 weeks with the aim to keep within reference range. Stabilize thyroid status on low dose of ATD/taper off ATDs before considering infertility treatments If RAI was chosen as a therapeutic option, wait for 6 months and for stable thyroid tests on LT4 replacement (TSH < 2.5 mIU/L on at least two occasions) before considering infertility treatment If surgery was chosen as a therapeutic option, wait till the patient has stable thyroid tests on LT4 replacement (TSH < 2.5 mIU/L on at least two occasions) before considering infertility treatment

Thyroid imbalance and male subfertility

In men, the influence of thyroid imbalance in fertility is less well established compared to women. There are few studies that have looked at this subject and are mainly association studies rather than observing the cause and effect relationship of thyroid dysfunction and subfertility. Thyroid dysfunction is associated with changes in SHBG that eventually impact the total and free testosterone levels.

Impact of hyperthyroidism and male subfertility

Hyperthyroidism leads to rise in SHBG and thus escalation in total testosterone levels.[65] Free testosterone is often reported to be normal in hyperthyroid men, but one study observed subnormal bioavailable testosterone in these men.[66] However, there is a lower free-testosterone-to-estradiol ratio in hyperthyroid men consequent to a higher total and free estradiol level and hence the higher incidence of gynecomastia and reduced libido in these men.[66] Hyperthyroidism impacts the hypothalamic–pituitary–testicular axis. The response of Leydig cells to exogenous administration of hCG is blunted as evident by testosterone levels.[67] In contrast, the gonadotropins (LH, FSH) show an exaggerated response to gonadotropin-releasing hormone (GnRH) administration.[67,68] These changes in hypothalamic–pituitary–testicular axis are reversible upon restitution of euthyroidism in these men. Semen abnormalities in terms of sperm count, motility, and morphology defects have been stated.[66,69] However, these findings are not consistent across studies, and on longitudinal follow-up, most of these defects improved as these men became euthyroid.[69] Hyperthyroidism adversely affects the sexual behavior, and increased prevalence of "hypoactive sexual desire (HSD)," "erectile dysfunction (ED)," "delayed ejaculation (DE)," and "premature ejaculation (PE)" is observed in different studies.[65,70] Mild ED is described in as much as 70% of hyperthyroid men compared to 34% in healthy controls.[71] This complaint of ED improves on achieving euthyroidism.[71] Investigators have studied the effect of radioactive iodine (RAI-131) treatment of hyperthyroidism on reproductive function. Only transient abnormalities if any were observed with relatively low doses of RAI-131 that are used to treat hyperthyroidism.[72] Even though no congenital anomalies or fetal loss in fathering a child within 3 months of RAI-131 has been observed, the ATA task force on radiation safety advises against attempting to produce pregnancy for at least 3 months after RAI-131 therapy.[73]

Impact of hypothyroidism and male subfertility

Compared to women, men have a low prevalence of hypothyroidism.[74,75] In contrast to hyperthyroidism, hypothyroidism leads to a reduction in SHBG and total testosterone levels, and up till a 60% fall in free testosterone is observed in men with hypothyroidism.[65] However, their gonadotropin levels are normal, suggesting that primary hypothyroidism induces hypogonadotropic hypogonadism in these men.[65] This is further proven by the fact that these men have blunted gonadotropin response to exogenously administered GnRH but have an exaggerated testosterone response to hCG administration, suggesting that the principal defect is at hypothalamic–pituitary–testicular axis and not at the level of Leydig cells.[76] It is noteworthy that after thyroid hormone replacement, SHBG and free testosterone levels return to normal.[77] Hypothyroidism adversely affects the sexual behavior, and up till 64% occurrence of HSD, ED, and DE and 7% frequency of PE are observed in men with untreated hypothyroidism.[70] These clinical features reverse to normal on restoration to euthyroidism with thyroid hormone replacement.[71] Semen abnormalities in terms of sperm count, motility, and morphology defects have been observed in men with hypothyroidism, but the results are not consistent across different studies. Krassas et al. studied 25 hypothyroid and 15 euthyroid men and noted that sperm morphology significantly and motility to a lesser extent differed between both groups.[78] These defects improved on restoration to euthyroidism.[78] Teratozoospermia was observed in 22.7% of hypothyroid men in another study investigating sperm abnormalities in 28 men with preexisting thyroid dysfunction.[79] Still, other investigators did not find significant association between hypothyroidism and sperm abnormalities.[80,81] Among male partners of infertile couples, 7.4% had SCH.[80] Our group recently reported 38.7% SCH and 6.8% hypothyroidism in 160 men with altered sperm parameters compared to 4.6% SCH in 216 men with normal sperm parameters.[82] We studied 376 male partners of couples presenting with subfertility and observed that sperm count, motility, and morphology reduced from euthyroidism to SCH and hypothyroid states; the latter two, i.e., motility and morphology, showed significant association with changing thyroid status.[82] Limited evidence is available on association of TPOAb and male subfertility. Trummer et al. did not report any significant association of thyroid status with sperm abnormalities in 305 men undergoing evaluation of subfertility.[83] However, they reported positive TPOAb in 7.5% of their study subjects, which was suggestively greater in men with any sperm abnormality (6.7% vs 1.6%; $P=0.04$) and asthenozoospermia (7.2% vs 1.6%; $P=0.5$), in comparison with normal sperm parameters.[83] We observed reduced sperm motility ($P=0.004$) and morphology ($P=0.01$) in men with positive TPOAb.[82]

In summary, the understanding of association of thyroid imbalance with male subfertility is evolving. We are still awaiting to know the cause and effect relationship of thyroid imbalance and TAI with male subfertility. There is a need for more research evidence on this subject and the effect of treatment of thyroid imbalance on male subfertility. While the scientific evidence is still accumulating, it seems prudent to evaluate the thyroid status in men with altered sperm parameters and/or sexual dysfunction to offer referral/treatment if an imbalance is observed.

References

1. Krassas G, Pontikides N, Kaltsas T, Papadopoulou P, Batrinos M. Menstrual disturbances in thyrotoxicosis. *Clin Endocrinol (Oxf)*. 1994;40(5):641–644. https://doi.org/10.1111/j.1365-2265.1994.tb03016.x.

2. Nasir S, Khan MM, Ahmed S, Alam S, Ullah S. Role of thyroid dysfunction in infertile women with menstrual disturbances. *Gomal J Med Sci.* 2016;14:20–24.

3. Rahman R, Saeed M, Zia S, Jan F, Muzaffar S, Waheed A. Thyroid disorders; prevalence of thyroid disorders in primary infertile women of reproductive age. *Prof Med J.* 2019;26(1):101–108. https://doi.org/10.29309/TPMJ/2019.26.01.2614.

4. Krassas G, Pontikides N, Kaltsas T, et al. Disturbances of menstruation in hypothyroidism. *Clin Endocrinol (Oxf).* 1999;50(5):655–659. https://doi.org/10.1046/j.1365-2265.1999.00719.x.

5. Quintino-Moro A, Zantut-Wittmann D, Tambascia M, Machado H, Fernandes A. High prevalence of infertility among women with Graves' disease and Hashimoto's thyroiditis. *Int J Endocrinol.* 2014;2014:1–6. https://doi.org/10.1155/2014/982705.

6. Poppe K, Glinoer D, Van Steirteghem A, et al. Thyroid dysfunction and autoimmunity in infertile women. *Thyroid.* 2002;12(11):997–1001. https://doi.org/10.1089/105072502320908330.

7. Al-Jaroudi D, Yassin S, Al Enezi N, Kaddour O, Al-Badr A. Hypothyroidism among subfertile women. *Clin Exp Obstet Gynecol.* 2018;45(1):63–67.

8. Lincoln SR, Ke RW, Kutteh WH. Screening for hypothyroidism in infertile women. *J Reprod Med.* 1999;44(5):455–457.

9. Abalovich M, Mitelberg L, Allami C, et al. Subclinical hypothyroidism and thyroid autoimmunity in women with infertility. *Gynecol Endocrinol.* 2007;23(5):279–283. https://doi.org/10.1080/09513590701259542.

10. Bharti G, Singh K, Kumari R, Kumar U. Prevalence of hypothyroidism in subfertile women in a tertiary care centre in North India. *Int J Res Med Sci.* 2017;5(5):1777.

11. Arojoki M, Jokimaa V, Juuti A, Koskinen P, Irjala K, Anttila L. Hypothyroidism among infertile women in Finland. *Gynecol Endocrinol.* 2000;14(2):127–131. https://doi.org/10.3109/09513590009167671.

12. Orouji Jokar T, Fourman LT, Lee H, Mentzinger K, Fazeli PK. Higher TSH levels within the normal range are associated with unexplained infertility. *J Clin Endocrinol Metab.* 2018;103(2):632–639.

13. Vissenberg R, Manders VD, Mastenbroek S, et al. Pathophysiological aspects of thyroid hormone disorders/thyroid peroxidase autoantibodies and reproduction. *Hum Reprod Update.* 2015;21(3):378–387.

14. Kachuei M, Jafari F, Kachuei A, Keshteli A. Prevalence of autoimmune thyroiditis in patients with polycystic ovary syndrome. *Arch Gynecol Obstet.* 2011;285(3):853–856. https://doi.org/10.1007/s00404-011-2040-5.

15. Ott J, Aust S, Kurz C, et al. Elevated antithyroid peroxidase antibodies indicating Hashimoto's thyroiditis are associated with the treatment response in infertile women with polycystic ovary syndrome. *Fertil Steril.* 2010;94(7):2895–2897. https://doi.org/10.1016/j.fertnstert.2010.05.063.

16. Korevaar TI, Mínguez-Alarcón L, Messerlian C, et al. Association of thyroid function and autoimmunity with ovarian reserve in women seeking infertility care. *Thyroid.* 2018;28(10):1349–1358.

17. Rao M, Wang H, Zhao S, et al. Subclinical hypothyroidism is associated with lower ovarian reserve in women aged 35 years or older. *Thyroid.* 2020;30(1):95–105.

18. Karmon A, Batsis M, Chavarro J, Souter I. Preconceptional thyroid-stimulating hormone levels and outcomes of intrauterine insemination among euthyroid infertile women. Fertil Steril. 2015; 103(1):258–263.e1. doi:10.1016/j.fertnstert.2014.09.035.

19. Reh A, Danoff A, Grifo J. What is a normal thyroid stimulating hormone (TSH) level? Effects of stricter TSH thresholds on pregnancy outcomes after IVF. *Fertil Steril.* 2010;94(4):S188. https://doi.org/10.1016/j.fertnstert.2010.07.731.

20. Chai J, Yeung W, Lee C, Li H, Ho P, Ng H. Live birth rates following in vitro fertilization in women with thyroid autoimmunity and/or subclinical hypothyroidism. *Clin Endocrinol (Oxf).* 2013;80(1):122–127. https://doi.org/10.1111/cen.12220.

21. So S, Yamaguchi W, Murabayashi N, Miyano N, Tawara F. Effect of moderately increased thyroid-stimulating hormone levels and presence of thyroid antibodies on pregnancy among infertile women. *Reprod Med Biol.* 2020;19(1):82–88.

22. Fumarola A, Grani G, Romanzi D, et al. Thyroid function in infertile patients undergoing assisted reproduction. *Am J Reprod Immunol.* 2013;70(4):336–341. https://doi.org/10.1111/aji.12113.

23. Weghofer A, Himaya E, Kushnir V, Barad D, Gleicher N. The impact of thyroid function and thyroid autoimmunity on embryo quality in women with low functional ovarian reserve: a case-control study. *Reprod Biol Endocrinol.* 2015;13(1). https://doi.org/10.1186/s12958-015-0041-0.

24. Green K, Werner M, Franasiak J, Juneau C, Hong K, Scott R. Investigating the optimal preconception TSH range for patients undergoing IVF when controlling for embryo quality. *J Assist Reprod Genet.* 2015;32(10):1469–1476. https://doi.org/10.1007/s10815-015-0549-4.

25. Rahman A, Abbassy H, Abbassy A. Improved in vitro fertilization outcomes after treatment of subclinical hypothyroidism in infertile women. *Endocr Pract.* 2010;16(5):792–797. https://doi.org/10.4158/ep09365.or.

26. Kim C, Ahn J, Kang S, Kim S, Chae H, Kang B. Effect of levothyroxine treatment on in vitro fertilization and pregnancy outcome in infertile women with subclinical hypothyroidism undergoing in vitro fertilization/intracytoplasmic sperm injection. *Fertil Steril.* 2011;95(5):1650–1654. https://doi.org/10.1016/j.fertnstert.2010.12.004.

27. Cai Y, Zhong L, Guan J, et al. Outcome of in vitro fertilization in women with subclinical hypothyroidism. *Reprod Med Biol.* 2017;15(1):39.

28. Rao M, Zeng Z, Zhao S, Tang L. Effect of levothyroxine supplementation on pregnancy outcomes in women with subclinical hypothyroidism and thyroid autoimmunity undergoing in vitro fertilization/intracytoplasmic sperm injection: an updated meta-analysis of randomized controlled trials. *Reprod Med Biol.* 2018;16(1):92.

29. Rao M, Zeng Z, Zhou F, et al. Effect of levothyroxine supplementation on pregnancy loss and preterm birth in women with subclinical hypothyroidism and thyroid autoimmunity: a systematic review and meta-analysis. *Hum Reprod Update.* 2019;25(3):344–361.

30. Akhtar MA, Agrawal R, Brown J, Sajjad Y, Craciunas L. Thyroxine replacement for subfertile women with euthyroid autoimmune thyroid disease or subclinical hypothyroidism. *Cochrane Database Syst Rev.* 2019;(6). https://doi.org/10.1002/14651858.CD011009.pub2.

31. Scoccia B, Demir H, Fierro M, Kang Y, Winston N. In vitro fertilization pregnancy rates in levothyroxine-treated women with hypothyroidism compared to women without thyroid dysfunction disorders. *Thyroid.* 2012;22:631–636. 120216031931006 https://doi.org/10.1089/thy.2011-0343.

32. Busnelli A, Somigliana E, Benaglia L, Leonardi M, Ragni G, Fedele L. In vitro fertilization outcomes in treated hypothyroidism. *Thyroid.* 2013;23(10):1319–1325. https://doi.org/10.1089/thy.2013.0044.

33. Jølving LR, Larsen MD, Fedder J, Friedman S, Nørgård BM. The chance of a live birth after assisted reproduction in women with thyroid disorders. *Clin Epidemiol.* 2019;11:683–694.

34. Chen CW, Huang YL, Tzeng CR, Huang RL, Chen CH. Idiopathic low ovarian reserve is associated with more frequent positive thyroid peroxidase antibodies. *Thyroid.* 2017;27(9):1194–1200.

35. Toulis K, Goulis D, Venetis C, et al. Risk of spontaneous miscarriage in euthyroid women with thyroid autoimmunity undergoing IVF: a meta-analysis. *Eur J Endocrinol.* 2010;162(4):643–652. https://doi.org/10.1530/eje-09-0850.

36. Tan S, Dieterle S, Pechlavanis S, Janssen O, Fuhrer D. Thyroid autoantibodies per se do not impair intracytoplasmic sperm injection outcome in euthyroid healthy women. *Eur J Endocrinol.* 2014;170(4):495–500. https://doi.org/10.1530/eje-13-0790.

37. Łukaszuk K, Kunicki M, Kulwikowska P, et al. The impact of the presence of antithyroid antibodies on pregnancy outcome following intracytoplasmatic sperm injection-ICSI and embryo transfer in women with normal thyreotropine levels. *J Endocrinol Invest.* 2015;38(12):1335–1343. https://doi.org/10.1007/s40618-015-0377-5.

38. Karacan M, Alwaeely F, Cebi Z, et al. Effect of antithyroid antibodies on ICSI outcome in antiphospholipid antibody-negative euthyroid women. *Reprod Biomed Online.* 2013;27(4):376–380. https://doi.org/10.1016/j.rbmo.2013.07.002.

39. Unuane D, Velkeniers B, Bravenboer B, et al. Impact of thyroid autoimmunity in euthyroid women on live birth rate after IUI. *Hum Reprod.* 2017;32(4):915–922.

40. Tuncay G, Karaer A, Coşkun Eİ, Baloğlu D, Tecellioğlu AN. The impact of thyroid-stimulating hormone levels in euthyroid women on intrauterine insemination outcome. *BMC Womens Health.* 2018;18(1):51.

41. Turgay B, Şükür YE, Ulubaşoğlu H, et al. The association of thyroid stimulating hormone levels and intrauterine insemination outcomes of euthyroid unexplained subfertile couples. *Eur J Obstet Gynecol Reprod Biol.* 2019;240:99–102.

42. Zhong Y, Ying Y, Wu H, et al. Relationship between antithyroid antibody and pregnancy outcome following in vitro fertilization and embryo transfer. *Int J Med Sci.* 2012;9(2):121–125. https://doi.org/10.7150/ijms.3467.

43. Medenica S, Garalejic E, Arsic B, et al. Follicular fluid thyroid autoantibodies, thyrotropin, free thyroxine levels and assisted reproductive technology outcome. *PLoS One.* 2018;13(10), e0206652.

44. Monteleone P, Parrini D, Faviana P, et al. Female infertility related to thyroid autoimmunity: the ovarian follicle hypothesis. *Am J Reprod Immunol.* 2011;66(2):108–114. https://doi.org/10.1111/j.1600-0897.2010.00961.x.

45. Cai YY, Lin N, Zhong LP, et al. Serum and follicular fluid thyroid hormone levels and assisted reproductive technology outcomes. *Reprod Biol Endocrinol.* 2019;17(1):90.

46. Litwicka K, Arrivi C, Varricchio M, Mencacci C, Greco E. In women with thyroid autoimmunity, does low-dose prednisolone administration, compared with no adjuvant therapy, improve in vitro fertilization clinical results? *J Obstet Gynaecol Res.* 2014;41(5):722–728. https://doi.org/10.1111/jog.12615.

47. Turi A, Giannubilo S, Zanconi S, Mascetti A, Tranquilli A. Preconception steroid treatment in infertile women with antithyroid autoimmunity undergoing ovarian stimulation and intrauterine insemination: a double-blind, randomized, prospective cohort study. *Clin Ther.* 2010;32(14):2415–2421. https://doi.org/10.1016/j.clinthera.2011.01.010.

48. Michael A, Papageorghiou A. Potential significance of physiological and pharmacological glucocorticoids in early pregnancy. *Hum Reprod Update.* 2008;14(5):497–517. https://doi.org/10.1093/humupd/dmn021.

49. Alexander EK, Pearce EN, Brent GA, et al. 2017 Guidelines of the American Thyroid Association for the diagnosis and management of thyroid disease during pregnancy and the postpartum. *Thyroid.* 2017;27(3):315–389.

50. Negro R, Mangieri T, Coppola L, et al. Levothyroxine treatment in thyroid peroxidase antibody-positive women undergoing assisted reproduction technologies: a prospective study. *Hum Reprod.* 2005;20(6):1529–1533. https://doi.org/10.1093/humrep/deh843.

51. Revelli A, Casano S, Piane L, et al. A retrospective study on IVF outcome in euthyroid patients with anti-thyroid antibodies: effects of levothyroxine, acetyl salicylic acid and prednisolone adjuvant treatments. *Reprod Biol Endocrinol.* 2009;7(1):137. https://doi.org/10.1186/1477-7827-7-137.

52. Wang H, Gao H, Chi H, et al. Effect of levothyroxine on miscarriage among women with normal thyroid function and thyroid autoimmunity undergoing in vitro fertilization and embryo transfer: a randomized clinical trial. *JAMA.* 2017;318(22):2190–2198.

53. Dhillon-Smith RK, Middleton LJ, Sunner KK, et al. Levothyroxine in women with thyroid peroxidase antibodies before conception. *N Engl J Med.* 2019;380:1316–1325. https://doi.org/10.1056/NEJMoa1812537.

54. Poppe K, Unuane D, D'Haeseleer M, et al. Thyroid function after controlled ovarian hyperstimulation in women with and without the hyperstimulation syndrome. *Fertil Steril.* 2011;96(1):241–245. https://doi.org/10.1016/j.fertnstert.2011.04.039.

55. Muller A, Verhoeff A, Mantel M, de Jong F, Berghout A. Decrease of free thyroxine levels after controlled ovarian hyperstimulation. *J Clin Endocrinol Metab.* 2000;85(2):545–548. https://doi.org/10.1210/jcem.85.2.6374.

56. Poppe K, Glinoer D, Tournaye H, et al. Impact of ovarian hyperstimulation on thyroid function in women with and without thyroid autoimmunity. *J Clin Endocrinol Metab.* 2004;89(8):3808–3812. https://doi.org/10.1210/jc.2004-0105.

57. Poppe K, Glinoer D, Tournaye H, Schiettecatte J, Haentjens P, Velkeniers B. Thyroid function after assisted reproductive technology in women free of thyroid disease. *Fertil Steril.* 2005;83(6):1753–1757. https://doi.org/10.1016/j.fertnstert.2004.12.036.

58. Gracia C, Morse C, Chan G, et al. Thyroid function during controlled ovarian hyperstimulation as part of in vitro fertilization. *Fertil Steril.* 2012;97(3):585–591. https://doi.org/10.1016/j.fertnstert.2011.12.023.

59. Reinblatt S, Herrero B, Correa J, et al. Thyroid stimulating hormone levels rise after assisted reproductive technology. *J Assist Reprod Genet.* 2013;30(10):1347–1352. https://doi.org/10.1007/s10815-013-0081-3.

60. Du YJ, Xin X, Cui N, et al. Effects of controlled ovarian stimulation on thyroid stimulating hormone in infertile women. *Eur J Obstet Gynecol Reprod Biol.* 2019;234:207–212.

61. Jin L, Wang M, Yue J, Zhu GJ, Zhang B. Association between TSH level and pregnancy outcomes in euthyroid women undergoing IVF/ICSI: a retrospective study and meta-analysis. *Curr Med Sci.* 2019;39(4):631–637.

62. Negro R. Thyroid and assisted reproduction technologies: a brief clinical update with recommendations for practice. *Endocr Metab Immune Disord Drug Targets.* 2018;18(3):194–200.

63. Stuckey B, Yeap D, Turner S. Thyroxine replacement during super-ovulation for in vitro fertilization: a potential gap in management? *Fertil Steril.* 2010;93(7):2414.e1–2414.e3. https://doi.org/10.1016/j.fertnstert.2009.11.051.

64. Busnelli A, Somigliana E, Benaglia L, Sarais V, Ragni G, Fedele L. Thyroid axis dysregulation during in vitro fertilization in hypothyroid-treated patients. *Thyroid.* 2014;24(11):1650–1655. https://doi.org/10.1089/thy.2014.0088.

65. Meikle A. The interrelationships between thyroid dysfunction and hypogonadism in men and boys. *Thyroid.* 2004;14(suppl. 1):17–25. https://doi.org/10.1089/105072504323024552.

66. Abalovich M, Levalle O, Hermes R, et al. Hypothalamic-pituitary-testicular axis and seminal parameters in hyperthyroid males. *Thyroid.* 1999;9(9):857–863. https://doi.org/10.1089/thy.1999.9.857.

67. Krassas G, Pontikides N. Male reproductive function in relation with thyroid alterations. *Best Pract Res Clin Endocrinol Metab.* 2004;18(2):183–195. https://doi.org/10.1016/j.beem.2004.03.003.

68. Zähringer S, Tomova A, von Werder K, Brabant G, Kumanov P, Schopohl J. The influence of hyperthyroidism on the hypothalamic-pituitary-gonadal axis. *Exp Clin Endocrinol Diabetes.* 2000;108(4):282–289. https://doi.org/10.1055/s-2000-7756.

69. Krassas G, Pontikides N, Deligianni V, Miras K. A prospective controlled study of the impact of hyperthyroidism on reproductive function in males. *J Clin Endocrinol Metab.* 2002;87(8):3667–3671. https://doi.org/10.1210/jcem.87.8.8714.

70. Carani C, Isidori A, Granata A, et al. Multicenter study on the prevalence of sexual symptoms in male hypo- and hyperthyroid patients. *J Clin Endocrinol Metab.* 2005;90(12):6472–6479. https://doi.org/10.1210/jc.2005-1135.

71. Krassas G, Tziomalos K, Papadopoulou F, Pontikides N, Perros P. Erectile dysfunction in patients with hyper- and hypothyroidism: how common and should we treat? *J Clin Endocrinol Metab.* 2008;93(5):1815–1819. https://doi.org/10.1210/jc.2007-2259.

72. Ceccarelli C, Canale D, Battisti P, et al. Testicular function after 131I therapy for hyperthyroidism. *Clin Endocrinol (Oxf).* 2006;65(4):446–452. https://doi.org/10.1111/j.1365-2265.2006.02613.x.

73. Sisson T, Freitas J, McDougall I, et al. Radiation safety in the treatment of patients with thyroid diseases by radioiodine 131I: practice recommendations of the American Thyroid Association. *Thyroid.* 2011;21(4):335–346. https://doi.org/10.1089/thy.2010.0403.

74. Bjoro T, Holmen J, Kruger O, et al. Prevalence of thyroid disease, thyroid dysfunction and thyroid peroxidase antibodies in a large, unselected population. The Health Study of Nord-Trondelag (HUNT). *Eur J Endocrinol.* 2000;143(5):639–647. https://doi.org/10.1530/eje.0.1430639.

75. Unnikrishnan A, Bantwal G, John M, Kalra S, Sahay R, Tewari N. Prevalence of hypothyroidism in adults: an epidemiological study in eight cities of India. *Indian J Endocrinol Metab.* 2013;17(4):647. https://doi.org/10.4103/2230-8210.113755.

76. Velázquez E, Arata G. Effects of thyroid status on pituitary gonadotropin and testicular reserve in men. *Arch Androl.* 1997;38(1):85–92. https://doi.org/10.3109/01485019708988535.

77. Donnelly P, White C. Testicular dysfunction in men with primary hypothyroidism; reversal of hypogonadotrophic hypogonadism with replacement thyroxine. *Clin Endocrinol (Oxf).* 2000;52(2):197–201. https://doi.org/10.1046/j.1365-2265.2000.00918.x.

78. Krassas G, Papadopoulou F, Tziomalos K, Zeginiadou T, Pontikides N. Hypothyroidism has an adverse effect on human spermatogenesis: a prospective, controlled study. *Thyroid.* 2008;18(12):1255–1259. https://doi.org/10.1089/thy.2008.0257.

79. Niroomand H, Binaafar S, Nasiri M, Mansournia N, Bagheri Behzad A. Sperm abnormalities: adverse effects of thyroid dysfunction. *J Basic Res Med Sci.* 2018;5(1):47–50. https://doi.org/10.29252/jbrms.5.1.47.

80. Lotti F, Maseroli E, Fralassi N, et al. Is thyroid hormones evaluation of clinical value in the work-up of males of infertile couples? *Hum Reprod.* 2016;31(3):518–529. https://doi.org/10.1093/humrep/dev338.

81. Poppe K, Glinoer D, Tournaye H, Maniewski U, Haentjens P, Velkeniers B. Is systematic screening for thyroid disorders indicated in subfertile men? *Eur J Endocrinol.* 2006;154(3):363–366. https://doi.org/10.1530/eje.1.02098.

82. Rehman R, Zafar A, Fatima SS, Mohib A, Sheikh A. Altered sperm parameters and subclinical hypothyroidism; a cross sectional study in Karachi, Pakistan. *Int J Clin Pract.* 2020. https://doi.org/10.1111/ijcp.13555.

83. Trummer H, Ramschak-Schwarzer S, Haas J, Habermann H, Pummer K, Leb G. Thyroid hormones and thyroid antibodies in infertile males. *Fertil Steril.* 2001;76(2):254–257. https://doi.org/10.1016/s0015-0282(01)01875-1.

Pituitary disorders and subfertility

10

Ishrat Khan[a,b] and Bhagwan Das[c]

[a]Consultant Diabetes & Endocrinology, Aneurin Bevan Health Board, Ysbyty Ystrad Fawr Hospital, Ystrad Mynach, United Kingdom, [b]Post Graduate Honorary Lecturer, Cardiff University and University of South Wales, Cardiff, United Kingdom, [c]Consultant Physician and Endocrinologist, Cancer Foundation Hospital, Karachi, Pakistan

Chapter outline

Introduction

The pituitary gland, also called the master gland of the human endocrine system, is situated at the base of the skull within the sella turcica, a part of the sphenoid bone. Anatomically it is divided into two parts: (i) the anterior part, also called adenohypophysis, and (ii) the posterior part, also called neurohypophysis. The adenohypophysis part works closely with the hypothalamus to control the function of other glands including gonads.

Gonadotropin-releasing hormone (GnRH) is released from hypothalamus periodically in pulses to control the secretion of two gonadotrophin hormones, luteinizing hormone (LH) and follicle-stimulating hormone (FSH). Both control functions and maturation of reproductive organs as shown in Fig. 10.1.

Subfertility. https://doi.org/10.1016/B978-0-323-75945-8.00010-4

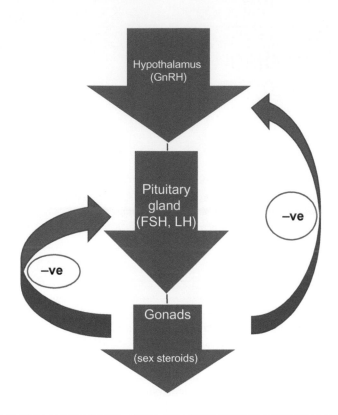

FIG. 10.1

Schematic diagram of hypothalamic–pituitary–gonadal axis.

The hypothalamic–pituitary–gonadal axis (HPGA) plays a fundamental role in fertility, and any disorder affecting pituitary, being a central position in this axis, can cause fertility issues. HPGA can be altered by many factors including congenital and acquired causes as mentioned in Table 10.1.[1,2]

Disorders of women ovulation are among the common causes of subfertility and are classified by WHO into three groups.[3] Approximately 10% of ovulatory disorders are secondary to HPGA defects and are categorized into group I. Group II constitutes around 85% of ovulatory disorders with normogonadotropic anovulation with predominantly polycystic ovaries, and group III includes disorders because of ovarian failure leading to hypergonadotropic hypogonadism.

A pituitary etiology should be considered in all patients whom initial workup points toward hypogonadotropic hypogonadism, i.e., low LH, FSH, and testosterone (Te)/estradiol (E2), or hyperprolactinemia. Most of these pituitary disorders are simple to manage medically with very good outcomes.

Table 10.1 Pituitary disorders that can result in subfertility.

A. Pituitary adenomas:
- o Functioning pituitary adenomas:
- o Prolactinoma, acromegaly, Cushing's disease
- o Nonfunctioning pituitary adenomas

B. Infarction:
- o Sheehan's syndrome
- o Pituitary apoplexy

C. Infiltrative lesions:
- o Hemochromatosis
- o Sarcoidosis
- o Hypophysitis
- o Histiocytosis

D. Infections:
- o Tuberculosis
- o Fungal infections
- o Abscess

E. Iatrogenic:
- o Pituitary surgery
- o Radiation

F. Empty sella

Approach to patients with subfertility

After a detailed history and examination, a preliminary workup in women with subfertility—but with regular cycles—is required to determine about their ovulation status by measuring serum progesterone levels during the midluteal phase (day 21). Serum progesterone with a level of ≥ 30 nmol/L is required to confirm the ovulation.[3,4] In women with no ovulation, serum progesterone level < 10 nmol/L or with irregular cycles, amenorrhea or oligomenorrhea, a further hormonal workup to assess the FSH, LH, E2, TSH, and serum prolactin is required to determine the underlying cause of subfertility.

In men with subfertility, following a detailed history and examination, the foremost step is to obtain seminal fluid analysis. Semen sample should be collected with an abstinence of 2–5 days from ejaculation. At least two samples on two different days, preferably 1 week apart,[5] are required, because of day-to-day variation in sperm concentrations.[6,7] A further hormonal workup—morning Te, FSH, LH, TSH, and prolactin—is required in case of abnormal semen analysis.

Separate investigations for acromegaly and Cushing's disease (CD) are required which would be disease specific, in addition to above initial subfertility work up. Magnetic resonance imaging (MRI) of the hypothalamic–pituitary region is mandatory in all cases with hypogonadotropic hypogonadism, pathological hyperprolactinemia, acromegaly, and CD.

Hyperprolactinemia and prolactinomas

Prolactin is a polypeptide hormone produced and secreted by the lactotroph cells of the anterior pituitary gland. In addition to its primary function of promoting lactation and breast development, it is associated with the reproductive system, immune system, behavioral changes, and also contributes to salt and water balance in the human body.[8] Its secretion is controlled by various hormones and neurotransmitters through tonic inhibition by dopamine.

Hyperprolactinemia means a higher level of prolactin in the blood above the normal reference range. Usually, normal reference range for prolactin level is between 10 and 35 ng/mL, with a conversion factor of 1 ng/mL = 21.2766 µIU/mL.[9] Hyperprolactinemia is a common disorder present in around 1% of the general population and 9%–17% of women with gonadal dysfunction.[10] Causes of hyperprolactinemia vary from idiopathic, physiological, and pharmacological to pathological as described in Table 10.2.[11–14]

Prolactinomas are the benign tumor of pituitary lactotroph cells. These are the most common functioning pituitary adenomas with an estimated prevalence of 45 cases/100,000 population.[15] They are more common in women with a women-to-men ratio of around 8:1, especially during reproductive age. In women, they are mostly microadenomas due to their early presentation with menstrual irregularities or galactorrhea, whereas in men, they present late and mostly have macroadenomas with hypogonadism.

Fertility and reproductive function in hyperprolactinemia

Hyperprolactinemia is frequently found in infertile women compared to fertile women with a prevalence of around 48%–51.7% in infertile women[16,17] and up to 11% in infertile men.[18] A high level of prolactin is associated with inhibition of

Table 10.2 Causes of hyperprolactinemia.

A. Idiopathic
B. Physiological:
  o Pregnancy, postpartum, lactation, sexual intercourse, stress, exercise, sleep, major surgery
C. Pathological:
  o Prolactinoma, acromegaly, nonfunctional pituitary adenoma, primary hypothyroidism, chest wall injury/herpes zoster infection, hepatic failure, renal failure, polycystic ovaries syndrome, seizures, pituitary infiltrative/infective diseases (Table 10.1)
D. Drug induced:
  o **Antidepressants:** Monoamine oxidase inhibitors, selective serotonin reuptake inhibitors, tricyclic antidepressants
  o **Antipsychotics:** Phenothiazine, haloperidol, risperidone
  o **Antihypertensive:** Verapamil, methyldopa, reserpine, tetrabenazine, labetalol
  o **Gastrointestinal medications:** Domperidone, metoclopramide, levosulpiride, proton pump inhibitors, H2 receptor blockers
  o **Miscellaneous:** Estrogen, opiates, cocaine, morphine, anesthetic, apomorphine, methadone

GnRH secretion from the hypothalamus and the low secretion of LH and FSH from pituitary gland.[19] In addition to hypothalamic–pituitary effect, high prolactin has direct gonadal effects at several other levels including ovarian estrogen production, maturation of follicles, ovulation, luteinization, and functioning of corpus luteum.[20–22] In men, it has a direct effect on Te production and spermatogenesis via prolactin receptors expressed on Leydig and Sertoli cells.[23,24]

These effects result in low estrogen and Te; thus, in women, it can present with amenorrhea, galactorrhea, decreased libido, and subfertility, while in men, it can present with decreased libido, erectile dysfunction, subfertility, gynecomastia, and rarely galactorrhea.

Because of long-term anovulation and an insufficient luteal phase observed in these women, hyperprolactinemia has been associated with defects in endometrial growth along with a failure of implantation.[25] In men, serum prolactin has been studied to have an inverse correlation with the sperm count.[26]

Management

After a detailed medical history and examination that focuses on all causes of hyperprolactinemia (Table 10.2), a further workup should be done to exclude other causes of hyperprolactinemia. The MRI of the hypothalamic–pituitary region is mandatory in all cases of hyperprolactinemia in which no obvious cause is identified.[11] Treatment is indicated in all symptomatic patients with hyperprolactinemia if even no lesion is identified on initial MRI or in patients with macroadenomas on MRI.

Treatment goals for the patients with prolactinomas are the normalization of serum prolactin level, decrease in the size of pituitary adenoma to reduce mass effects, restoration of gonadal dysfunction, and fertility.

Dopamine agonists (DAs) are the most effective treatment option in patients with prolactinomas by reducing the prolactin levels, thus restoring gonadal dysfunction and fertility issues. Cabergoline is preferred over bromocriptine because of its better efficacy, convenient dosage, and better tolerability. In one of the largest follow-up studies of 459 women with hyperprolactinemic amenorrhea, resolution of the ovulatory cycle or pregnancy was reported in 72% of the women who were managed with cabergoline and 52% of the women who were managed with bromocriptine.[27] Because of its shorter half-life and relatively a safer option, bromocriptine is preferred over cabergoline for pregnancy induction.

In patients with microadenomas, after normalization of prolactin and restoration of ovulation, pregnancy is usually delayed for up to three to four regular menstrual cycles, time sufficient to predict pregnancy in case of any missed cycle. While in patients with macroadenomas, pregnancy is usually delayed until the size of the tumor decreased to microadenoma or it becomes confined to sella, so that they do not have to continue DAs during pregnancy.

In those patients, who do not ovulate despite normalization of prolactin levels, cyclical administration of clomiphene citrate, gonadotropins, or pulsatile GnRH can be combined with DAs to increase the success rates of fertility.

Acromegaly

Acromegaly is a rare chronic multisystemic disorder of pituitary origin, with an incidence of 0.2–1.1 cases per 100,000 population with an estimated prevalence of 2.8–13.7 cases per 100,00 population annually.[28] In most of the cases, it is caused by growth hormone (GH) secreting pituitary adenoma with an equal ratio in men and women. In a few cases, it can result from ectopic GH secretion or secondary to growth hormone-releasing hormone adenoma of hypothalamic origin. Because of its insidious onset, it is usually diagnosed around the age of 40, with a delay of 4–5 years after the disease onset.[28]

Fertility and reproductive function in acromegaly

Gonadal dysfunction is a common clinical entity in both sexes[29] with acromegaly and has been reported in around 59%–70% of women with this condition,[30,31] while in data on men, information regarding this effect is lacking. Hypogonadism in patients with acromegaly can be explained by various mechanisms, these include anatomical compression of HPGA by mass effect, hyperprolactinemia caused by GH and prolactin cosecretion, or by dopamine inhibition by stalk compression. The lactotrophic effect of GH (spillover effect) may influence gonadal dysfunction.

In addition to these effects, recent data suggest that GH and insulin-like growth factor 1 (IGF-1) have also a direct inhibitory effect over ovarian function.[30] IGF-1 locally increases androgen production from theca cells of ovarian follicles,[32] resulting in hyperandrogenemia and polycystic ovarian morphology along with menstrual irregularities.[33]

In one study on men with acromegaly, it was found that serum Te was below normal in 42.8%, and dihydrotestosterone (DHT) was low in 65.7% along with low seminal volume, total sperm count, sperm count per mL, normal morphology, vitality, total motility, and forward progression.[34]

Spontaneous pregnancy in untreated patients is very rare, less than 158 reported in the literature.[35,36] With the advancement in surgical, medical, and reproductive techniques, pregnancies have been reported more frequently than before in this group of patients.[37]

Women with this condition, who want to get pregnant, should be advised to undergo treatment of acromegaly first to avoid the expansion of pituitary adenoma before pregnancy, normalization of hyperprolactinemia, GH, and IGF-1 levels to maximize their fertility potential. They should also be assessed for the deficiency of other pituitary hormones and should be adequately replaced before undergoing any fertility treatment.

Men with the condition, after treatment and normalization of GH/IGF-1 levels, have been reported to show an improvement in Te and DHT levels with an increase in the volume of the semen along with an improvement in other parameters such as sperm count and motility.[34]

Cushing's disease

CD is a rare endocrine disorder of the pituitary origin characterized by chronic hypercortisolemia. The incidence of CD is 1.2–2.4/million population per year with an estimated prevalence of around 40 cases/million population.[38,39] CD is more common among women and is mostly diagnosed during the age of 40–60 years, thus rarely encountered in the fertility clinics.

Fertility and reproductive function in Cushing's disease

Hypercortisolemia can affect the reproductive system, resulting in menstrual irregularities in more than two-thirds of women with this condition.[40] Most of the women with CD present clinically with similar signs and symptoms that are observed in young women with PCOS, irregular cycles, hirsutism, acne, obesity, hyperandrogenism, low SHBG levels, and an increased gonadotropin response to GnRH.[41,42]

Hypogonadism in patients with CD can be explained by various mechanisms, such as inhibition of HPGA by both chronic hypercortisolemia and adrenal hyperandrogenism and also by high levels of adrenocorticotropic hormone and corticotropin-releasing hormone, resulting in low levels of LH and estrogen and thus chronic anovulation. In addition, ovaries in CD have been reported to have decreased size, a low number of follicles, absence of luteinization, and fibrosis.[43]

In men, information regarding the effects of CD on testicular function is very limited and thought to be due to sparse Leydig cells, the thickened basement of seminiferous tubules, and low spermatogenesis on histology.[44] If patients have macroadenoma, hypogonadism and fertility may further be affected by hyperprolactinemia due to stalk effect, though less common in CD as mostly they are associated with microadenoma.

Nonfunctioning pituitary adenomas

Nonfunctioning pituitary adenomas (NFPAs) is the second most common cause of pituitary adenoma after prolactinomas with an estimated prevalence of 7–41.3 cases/100,000 population.[45] NFPAs are rare during reproductive age as their peak occurrence has been reported between 40 and 80 years.[45]

NFPAs do not have any hormonal activity and are thus detected clinically late with symptoms, such as headaches, visual defects, cranial nerve palsies, and hormonal deficiencies. Endocrine manifestations of NFPAs depend upon the size and degree of compression by NFPAs over normal pituitary tissues.[46] They can present clinically with a varying degree of hormonal deficiencies from partial hypopituitarism (37%–85%) to panhypopituitarism (6%–29%).[45]

Hypogonadotropic hypogonadism is one of the common hormonal deficiencies in around 38%–72% of patients with clinical symptoms of low libido, erectile dysfunction, and disorders of menstruation.[47,48] Hyperprolactinemia observed in NFPAs is usually mild and occurs because of blockage of dopaminergic inhibition of lactotroph by pituitary adenoma, called a stalk effect.

During a normal pregnancy, pituitary size is expected to increase by an average of 120% with a 40% increase in lactotrophs.[49,50] The effect of pregnancy on the actual size of NFPAs is a less expected phenomenon, though lactotrophic hyperplasia can present with chiasmal compression. Due to advances in the treatment of pituitary tumors and subfertility, many women are getting pregnant with pituitary disorders. In recently reported two case series, 23 cases of NFPAs have been reported in pregnancies with good pregnancy outcomes but with an increased rate of cesarean section deliveries than controls.[51,52]

Summary

The management of subfertility in patients with pituitary disorders requires shared care by endocrinologists, neurosurgeons, and fertility specialists. Prolactinomas are the most common pituitary disorders linked with subfertility, with a positive outcome in most cases with the appropriate treatment. For other causes of subfertility such as acromegaly and CD requires management of underlying disease itself as surgical removal of adenoma for rapid restoration of endocrine dysfunction and fertility outcomes. Medical therapy is usually discontinued upon confirmation of pregnancy with close monitoring of signs and symptoms of compression throughout the pregnancy. In patients with NFPAs, adequate hormonal replacement is the aim to preserve fertility along with monitoring for new hormone deficiencies and increase in thyroid hormones and glucocorticoids requirements during pregnancy.

References

1. Deep J. Assisted reproductive technology. *J Chitwan Med Coll.* 2014;4.
2. Ibrahim A, Othman M, Afendi N. *A Quick Guide to the Management of Infertility.* School of Medical Sciences; 2011.
3. National Collaborating Centre for Women's & Children's Health. National Institute for Health and Clinical Excellence: Guidance. *Fertility: Assessment and Treatment for People With Fertility Problems.* London: Royal College of Obstetricians & Gynaecologists Copyright © 2013, National Collaborating Centre for Women's and Children's Health; 2013.
4. Li RH, Ng EH. Management of anovulatory infertility. *Best Pract Res Clin Obstet Gynaecol.* 2012;26(6):757–768.
5. Agarwal A, Gupta S, Du Plessis S, et al. Abstinence time and its impact on basic and advanced semen parameters. *Urology.* 2016;94:102–110.
6. Jungwirth A, Giwercman A, Tournaye H, et al. European association of urology guidelines on male infertility: the 2012 update. *Eur Urol.* 2012;62(2):324–332.
7. Male Infertility Best Practice Policy Committee of the American Urological Association; Practice Committee of the American Society for Reproductive Medicine. Report on optimal evaluation of the infertile male. *Fertil Steril.* 2006;86(5 suppl. 1):S202–S209.
8. Freeman ME, Kanyicska B, Lerant A, Nagy G. Prolactin: structure, function, and regulation of secretion. *Physiol Rev.* 2000;80(4):1523–1631.
9. Davis JR. Prolactin and reproductive medicine. *Curr Opin Obstet Gynecol.* 2004;16(4):331–337.

10. Biller BM, Luciano A, Crosignani PG, et al. Guidelines for the diagnosis and treatment of hyperprolactinemia. *J Reprod Med.* 1999;44(12 suppl):1075–1084.
11. Melmed S, Casanueva FF, Hoffman AR, et al. Diagnosis and treatment of hyperprolactinemia: an Endocrine Society Clinical Practice Guideline. *J Clin Endocrinol Metabol.* 2011;96(2):273–288.
12. Demssie Y, Davis J. Hyperprolactinaemia. *Clin Med (Lond).* 2008;8:216–219.
13. Oner G. Prolactin and infertility. In: Nagy GM, Toth BE, eds. *Prolactin.* InTech; 2013:147–166.
14. Majumdar A, Mangal N. Hyperprolactinemia. *J Hum Reprod Sci.* 2013;6(3):168–175.
15. Lopes MBS. Pathology of prolactinomas: any predictive value? *Pituitary.* 2020;23(1):3–8.
16. Isah I, Aliyu I, Yusuf R, Isah H, Randawa A, Adesiyun A. Hyperprolactinemia and female infertility: pattern of clinical presentation in a tertiary health facility in Northern Nigeria. *Sahel Med J.* 2018;21(1):1–5.
17. Emokpae MA, Vadia PO, Mohammed AZ. Hormonal evaluations and endometrial biopsy in infertile women in Kano, Northern Nigeria: a comparative study. *Ann Afr Med.* 2005;4(3):99–103.
18. Singh P, Singh M, Cugati G, Singh A. Hyperprolactinemia: an often missed cause of male infertility. *J Hum Reprod Sci.* 2011;4(2):102.
19. Kaiser UB. Hyperprolactinemia and infertility: new insights. *J Clin Invest.* 2012;122(10):3467–3468.
20. Kauppila A, Martikainen H, Puistola U, Reinila M, Ronnberg L. Hypoprolactinemia and ovarian function. *Fertil Steril.* 1988;49(3):437–441.
21. Kauppila A, Leinonen P, Vihko R, Ylostalo P. Metoclopramide-induced hyperprolactinemia impairs ovarian follicle maturation and corpus luteum function in women. *J Clin Endocrinol Metab.* 1982;54(5):955–960.
22. Jacobs HS. Prolactin and amenorrhea. *N Engl J Med.* 1976;295(17):954–956.
23. Raut S, Deshpande S, Balasinor NH. Unveiling the role of prolactin and its receptor in male reproduction. *Horm Metab Res.* 2019;51(4):215–219.
24. Hair WM, Gubbay O, Jabbour HN, Lincoln GA. Prolactin receptor expression in human testis and accessory tissues: localization and function. *Mol Hum Reprod.* 2002;8(7):606–611.
25. Berkhout RP, Lambalk CB, Repping S, Hamer G, Mastenbroek S. Premature expression of the decidualization marker prolactin is associated with repeated implantation failure. *Gynecol Endocrinol.* 2019;1–5.
26. Adejuwon CA, Ilesanmi AO, Ode EO. Hyperprolactinaemia as a cause of male infertility in Ibadan. *West Afr J Med.* 1999;18(1):17–19.
27. Webster J, Piscitelli G, Polli A, Ferrari CI, Ismail I, Scanlon MF. A comparison of cabergoline and bromocriptine in the treatment of hyperprolactinemic amenorrhea. *N Engl J Med.* 1994;331(14):904–909.
28. Lavrentaki A, Paluzzi A, Wass JAH, Karavitaki N. Epidemiology of acromegaly: review of population studies. *Pituitary.* 2017;20(1):4–9.
29. Melmed S, Ho K, Klibanski A, Reichlin S, Thorner M. Clinical review 75: recent advances in pathogenesis, diagnosis, and management of acromegaly. *J Clin Endocrinol Metab.* 1995;80(12):3395–3402.
30. Grynberg M, Salenave S, Young J, Chanson P. Female gonadal function before and after treatment of acromegaly. *J Clin Endocrinol Metabol.* 2010;95(10):4518–4525.
31. Katznelson L, Kleinberg D, Vance ML, et al. Hypogonadism in patients with acromegaly: data from the multi-centre acromegaly registry pilot study. *Clin Endocrinol (Oxf).* 2001;54(2):183–188.
32. Chandrashekar V, Zaczek D, Bartke A. The consequences of altered somatotropic system on reproduction. *Biol Reprod.* 2004;71(1):17–27.

33. Kaltsas GA, Androulakis II, Tziveriotis K, et al. Polycystic ovaries and the polycystic ovary syndrome phenotype in women with active acromegaly. *Clin Endocrinol (Oxf)*. 2007;67(6):917–922.
34. Colao A, De Rosa M, Pivonello R, et al. Short-term suppression of GH and IGF-I levels improves gonadal function and sperm parameters in men with acromegaly. *J Clin Endocrinol Metabol*. 2002;87(9):4193–4197.
35. Cheng S, Grasso L, Martinez-Orozco JA, et al. Pregnancy in acromegaly: experience from two referral centers and systematic review of the literature. *Clin Endocrinol (Oxf)*. 2012;76(2):264–271.
36. Arefzadeha A, Shalbaf NA, Khalighinejadb P, Darvishzadeha A. Maternal and fetal effects of acromegaly on pregnancy. Clinical Practice and Drug Treatment. *Int J Adv Biotechnol Res*. 2016;7(3):952–960.
37. Laway BA. Pregnancy in acromegaly. *Ther Adv Endocrinol Metab*. 2015;6(6):267–272.
38. Fleseriu M, Hamrahian AH, Hoffman AR, Kelly DF, Katznelson L. American Association of Clinical Endocrinologists and American College of Endocrinology Disease State Clinical Review: diagnosis of recurrence in Cushing disease. *Endocr Pract*. 2016;22(12):1436–1448.
39. Steffensen C, Bak AM, Rubeck KZ, Jorgensen JO. Epidemiology of Cushing's syndrome. *Neuroendocrinology*. 2010;92(suppl. 1):1–5.
40. Lado-Abeal J, Rodriguez-Arnao J, Newell-Price JD, et al. Menstrual abnormalities in women with Cushing's disease are correlated with hypercortisolemia rather than raised circulating androgen levels. *J Clin Endocrinol Metab*. 1998;83(9):3083–3088.
41. Geer EB, Shafiq I, Gordon MB, et al. Biochemical control during long-term follow-up of 230 adult patients with cushing disease: a multicenter retrospective study. *Endocr Pract*. 2017;23(8):962–970.
42. Brzana J, Yedinak CG, Hameed N, Plesiu A, McCartney S, Fleseriu M. Polycystic ovarian syndrome and Cushing's syndrome: a persistent diagnostic quandary. *Eur J Obstet Gynecol Reprod Biol*. 2014;175:145–148.
43. Iannaccone A, Gabrilove JL, Sohval AR, Soffer LJ. The ovaries in Cushing's syndrome. *N Engl J Med*. 1959;261:775–780.
44. Jequier AM, ed. Endocrine infertility. In: *Male Infertility: A Clinical Guide. Cambridge Clinical Guides*. 2nd ed. Cambridge: Cambridge University Press; 2011:181–196.
45. Ntali G, Wass JA. Epidemiology, clinical presentation and diagnosis of non-functioning pituitary adenomas. *Pituitary*. 2018;21(2):111–118.
46. Mukai K, Kitamura T, Tamada D, Murata M, Otsuki M, Shimomura I. Relationship of each anterior pituitary hormone deficiency to the size of non-functioning pituitary adenoma in the hospitalized patients. *Endocr J*. 2016;63(11):965–976.
47. Molitch ME. Nonfunctioning pituitary tumors and pituitary incidentalomas. *Endocrinol Metab Clin North Am*. 2008;37(1):151–171. xi.
48. Ferrante E, Ferraroni M, Castrignanò T, et al. Non-functioning pituitary adenoma database: a useful resource to improve the clinical management of pituitary tumors. *Eur J Endocrinol*. 2006;155(6):823–829.
49. Laway BA, Mir SA. Pregnancy and pituitary disorders: challenges in diagnosis and management. *Indian J Endocrinol Metab*. 2013;17(6):996–1004.
50. Molitch ME. Pituitary diseases in pregnancy. *Semin Perinatol*. 1998;22(6):457–470.
51. Lambert K, Rees K, Seed PT, et al. Macroprolactinomas and nonfunctioning pituitary adenomas and pregnancy outcomes. *Obstet Gynecol*. 2017;129(1):185–194.
52. Karaca Z, Yarman S, Ozbas I, et al. How does pregnancy affect the patients with pituitary adenomas: a study on 113 pregnancies from Turkey. *J Endocrinol Invest*. 2018;41(1):129–141.

Oxidative stress and oocyte microenvironment

11

Faiza Alam

Clinical Academia, Pengiran Anak Puteri Rashidah Sa'adatul Bolkiah Institute of Health Science, Universiti Brunei Darussalam, Bandar Seri Begawan, Brunei

Chapter outline

Females inherit a reservoir of around 300,000 primordial follicles, with primary oocytes arrested at the first meiotic division. They attain maturation into the functional phase toward diversity periodically every month by regulators that govern them to survive or lead them toward apoptosis.[1,2] As a consequence, few attain completion and reach ovulation to be fertilized by male gametes.[3] In order to complete the development, a number of genetic, epigenetic, and cytoplasmic modifications occur before fertilization. Preservation of the ovarian pool is thus a very important factor that is subject to insult by a number of extrinsic and intrinsic factors.[4]

Redox environment of the ovaries

The free radical theory of aging implies that reactive chemical species are indispensable for the prevention of oxidative damage with increasing age,[5] leading to atresia of the follicles and aged oocytes.[6] Oxidative imbalance due to mitochondrial dysfunction may result in chromosomal segregation disorders, fertilization failures, formation of fragmented oocytes, and fragmentation of the embryos.[7,8] The normal

Subfertility. https://doi.org/10.1016/B978-0-323-75945-8.00011-6

mechanism of the male and female reproductive systems requires a controlled redox activity and an increase in reactive oxygen species (ROS) may lead to subfertility.[8]

Oxidant and antioxidant system

The moderate escalation of ROS acts favorably for oocyte maturity. Nevertheless, higher levels worsen the oocyte quality, thus impacting the reproductive capability.[6,8–10] Free radicals are continually released by the mitochondria during the process of energy production. The preservation of the oxidative environment is essential for the natural development of oocytes, cell integrity, and hormonal activities.[11] Free radical oxidation can contribute to follicular atresia and aged oocytes.[6]

OS and ovarian reserve

The increase in age and psychological stress are the two most important factors that influence the fertilizing capacity of the oocytes. With the approach of menopause, there is a decline of the ovarian reserve that affects the normal cyclic hormonal process and the functional capacity of the oocytes required for fertility.[12]

Effect of obesity on the microenvironment of the ovary

Reproductive potential decreases with increases in body weight. Obesity, an established risk factor for subfertility, develops resistance not only to insulin but also to gonadotropins, building an indirect role in oocyte capacity for its maturation and fertilization.[13] Obesity leads to subfertility by inflammation, mitochondrial dysfunction, and the disturbance of the hypothalamic–pituitary axis caused by increased androgen production in obese females, which may end in anovulation and menstrual irregularities. The resultant inflammation due to obesity in addition generates ROS, with a similar impact on the quality of oocytes.[14]

Stress and subfertility

Immense amounts of data support depression and anxiety as being responsible for impaired fecundity. Society renders females responsible for not bearing a child. Abnormal levels of stress markers such as adrenaline and cortisol have been recorded on the oocyte pickup day exhibiting high levels of anxiety in infertile females, unveiling the influence of stress on the hypothalamic–pituitary–adrenal (HPA) axis.[15] The disturbed redox environment and oxidative damage can instigate neurodegenerative diseases by apoptosis, excitotoxicity, and neuronal damage.[16,17] However, the impact of stress and anxiety on subfertility has yet to be proved.[18]

Reproductive hormones and OS

An increase in ROS has an inverse relationship with estradiol production affecting the ovarian response.[19] Due to OS, the disturbed levels of LH and FSH levels cause inadequate oocyte maturation, impaired fertilization, decreased cleavage, and pregnancy loss.[20,21]

Oxidative stress generation within oocytes

Relation of SIRT1 and subfertility

Sirtuins (NAD-dependent deacylases) are involved in deacetylation of histone and transcriptional factors affecting the protein and regulating the cell cycle. They play an important role in providing resistance to oxidation stress and regulating metabolism not only in the nucleus but also in the cytoplasm and mitochondria.[22,23] SIRT1 is a sensor and guardian of the redox state in female reproductive cells.[24] SIRT1 prevents damage to ovarian cells by the deacetylation of transcription factors such as forkhead-box (FOXO), which is accountable for the expression of superoxides.[25] The mitochondrial biogenesis raises the mitochondrial mass and controls glutathione peroxide, catalase, and manganese SOD by stimulating the peroxisome proliferator-activated receptor coactivator 1-α (PGc1a).[26,27]

SIRT1 catalyzes the enzymatic reaction between nicotinamide and the acetyl group of the substrate to form a metabolite O-acetyl ADP ribose by NAD cleavage, which positively affects ovarian cell growth.[28] The SIRT1 genotype regulates normal embryogenesis by controlling the proliferation and apoptosis of granulosa cells. In sirtuin-deficit mice, the phenotype is small with a congenital defect with postnatal death early in life.[29] SIRT1 increases ovarian hormones by maintaining the oxidative milieu in favor of the growth and maturation of the oocytes.[30]

Glucose homeostasis and insulin secretion are also regulated by SIRT1, as its function is to deacetylate PGC-1a, which is a main transcriptional coactivator regulating the hepatic glucose metabolism by gene transcription.[26] Animal studies show that SIRT1 upregulates insulin secretion in response to glucose stimulation, assisting glucose tolerance.[31] Furthermore, it reduces fat deposits in adipose tissues by suppressing PPARg and also aids in resolving obesity, indirectly lowering the intensity of insulin resistance and type 2 diabetes.[32]

PCOS patients are obese and display insulin resistance.[33] As postulated by some researchers, metformin helps reduce OS in PCOS patients by disturbing SIRT1.[34] Adipose tissue possesses a secretory capacity of angiotensin II, indirectly stimulating nicotinamide adenine dinucleotide phosphate (NADPH) oxidase activity and increasing ROS production in adipocytes.[35]

SIRT1 is an efficient antioxidant found in the oocyte, where it regulates energy production by the mitochondria.[36,37] Mitochondrial enzymes, including manganese superoxide dismutase (MnSOD), acting as antioxidants within the oocytes are deacylated by SIRT1.[38,39]

MnSOD plays a vital role in battling OS within an oocyte, probably by its posttranslational, posttranscriptional alteration.[40,41] SIRT1 activity also prevents an oxidant environment by dietary antioxidant approaches,[42] perhaps by modifying the energy expense and production.[43] MnSOD counterbalances negatively charged ions (O^{2-}) and finally converts them into soluble water (H_2O) inside the mitochondrial substance.[44]

SIRT1 mutations disturb the production of MnSOD in various tissues, including the granulosa cells and the oocytes, thus developing OS. Alteration in MnSOD levels is subject to SIRT1 genetic modification.[45,46] SIRT1 chiefly contributes in the course of oogenesis with its expression in the oocytes extending to the metaphase II phase (MII), as compared to the SIRT3, which takes part in fertilization and primary embryonic growth.[47] Thus, SIRT1 has a conventional participation in positively regulating the release of ovarian steroids.[36] Resveratrol acts as a broad-spectrum stimulator of SIRT1, which can be used to reduce OS and hence correct luteal defects in subfertile patients.[48]

Metformin is a hypoglycemic drug inhibiting the hepatic gluconeogenesis. In a dose-dependent fashion, it has the capability to inhibit cellular respiration within the mitochondria of hepatic cells by increasing the NAD^+/NADH ratio and SIRT1 activities. Metformin regulates glutathione content by employing cell-signaling mechanisms for mitochondrial regulation, hence improving OS[34,36,49,50] (see Fig. 11.1).

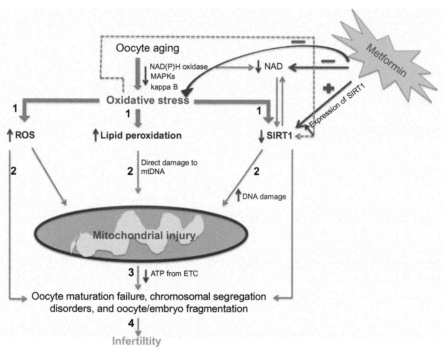

FIG. 11.1

A hypothetical interpretation of the probable mechanisms metformin adapts to maintain the microenvironment of the human granulosa cells. Advancing age induces oxidative stress in the oocytes, thus increasing lipid peroxidation and concurrently decreasing the expression of SIRT1 via a decreased NAD/NADPH ratio (STEP1). This causes a disturbance in the mitochondrial function by direct damage to the mitochondrial DNA (STEP2), reducing ATP synthesis by the electron transport chain (STEP3). Consequently, oocyte maturation failure, chromosomal segregation disorders, and oocyte/embryo fragmentation occur (STEP4), resulting in infertility. Metformin regulates the NAD/NADPH ratio indirectly and the expression of SIRT1 directly. ATP, adenosine-5-triphosphate; MAPKs, mitogen-activated protein kinase; mtDNA, mitochondrial DNA; NAD(P)H, nicotinamide adenine dinucleotide phosphate; ROS, reactive oxygen species; SIRT, sirtuin.[34]

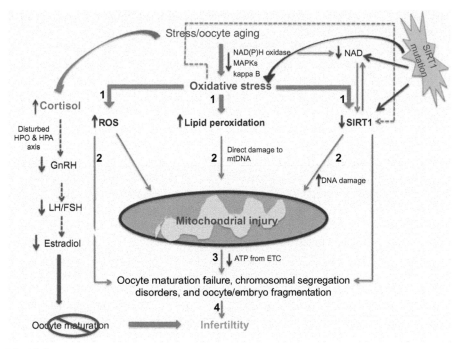

FIG. 11.2

Hypothetical illustration of SIRT1 and oocyte aging mechanism affecting the microenvironment. Advancing age induces oxidative stress in the oocytes, thus increasing lipid peroxidation and concurrently decreasing the expression of SIRT1 via a decreased NAD/NADPH ratio (STEP1). This causes a disturbance in the mitochondrial function by direct damage to the mitochondrial DNA (STEP2), reducing ATP synthesis by the electron transport chain (STEP3). Stress instigates the release of cortisol due to the HPO and HPA axis dysfunction. Consequently, oocyte maturation failure, chromosomal segregation disorders, and oocyte/embryo fragmentation occur (STEP4), resulting in infertility.

Metformin regulates SIRT1 by producing the cytokine visfatin, which takes part in NAD production, immune functions, and metabolic disorders (Fig. 11.2).[36]

Glutathione is another antioxidant within the oocyte and the embryo, where it functions as a reducing agent linked to the glucose metabolism.[51] Reduced NADH produced in the pentose phosphate pathway is imperative to keep glutathione in the reduced state.[52] The exhaustion of glutathione reductase can possibly increase hydrogen peroxide (H_2O_2) levels, which can potentially damage the DNA.[53] This effect of a decrease in glutathione levels can cause chromosomal aberrations and maturation failures of an oocyte. Cortisol levels increase with persistent psychological stress and with a combination of decreased GR, it is impossible to combat OS. Physical stress together with emotional stress can cause corticotropin-releasing hormone secretion, resulting in higher plasma cortisol levels.[54] Chronic stress also inhibits natural killer cell action along with the activity of T lymphocytes causing immunosuppression, which may lead to endometriosis and hormonal alterations compromising the formation of gamete and impairment of embryo development and implantation.[54]

The expression of visfatin in human ovarian follicles, follicular fluid, and granulosa-like tumor cell line (KGN) cells is regulated by metformin through SIRT1 signaling pathways.[55] Metformin induces a rise in the NAD^+/NADH ratio by activating the amplified appearance of visfatin, resulting in enhanced SIRT1 expression.[55] Visfatin positively effects the insulin-like growth factor-1-induced steroidogenesis in obese individuals. Visfatin revolves around SIRT1 expression and promotes steroidogenesis in the granulosa cells.[56] Visfatin increases in response to low-level antioxidants in obese individuals and its expression is negatively associated with the antioxidants produced.[57] Thus, visfatin is connected with the genes related to OS and the inflammatory responses,[58] which makes it a powerful contender among OS biomarkers, especially in newborns, for a better choice of treatment.[59]

Visfatin is synthesized in visceral adipose tissue and the ovarian follicles,[55,60,61] the myometrium,[62] and the placenta[63] of mammals. It plays a role in many metabolic reactions, inflammatory processes, and cellular energy production. SIRT1, being NAD-dependent deacetylase, requires visfatin to accomplish its metabolic goals.[64] Visfatin increases the insulin-like growth factor-induced steroidogenesis in the granulosa cells of humans[55] as well as gonadotropin production.[65] The literature supports the presence of increased levels of visfatin in type 2 diabetes and PCOS.[66]

Adrenaline

Adrenaline is a catecholamine neurotransmitter produced by the sympathetic nervous system and the adrenal medulla.[67] Pertaining to its connection with the oxidative environment, two potential consequences can be predicted. It can be involved in OS production as well as protection from OS. High levels of adrenaline and dopamine have been documented in the follicular fluid of PCOS.[68] Prolonged stress increases adrenaline production, which crosses the blood–brain barrier and disturbs the HPA axis with an increase in cortisol production due to an increase in the cortisol releasing factor.[54] An increased level of adrenaline is an attribute of obesity, as increased adipose tissues trigger sympathetic activity in females.[69]

Stress hormones, follicular size, and endometrial thickness

Conservation of the oxidative setting seems to indeed be required for the maturation of the follicles and endothelium; however, oxidants hamper the follicular maturity. Levels of oxidants and antioxidants are fairly different between individuals with an endometrial thickness cut-off of 0.8 mm and among those with a follicular size of 2 cm, more or less.

References

1. Craig J, Orisaka M, Wang H, et al. Gonadotropin and intra-ovarian signals regulating follicle development and atresia: the delicate balance between life and death. *Front Biosci.* 2006;12:3628–3639.
2. McGinnis LK, Limback SD, Albertini DF. Signaling modalities during oogenesis in mammals. *Curr Top Dev Biol.* 2012;102:227–242.

3. Sobinoff, A., Sutherland, J., & Mclaughlin, E. (2013). Intracellular signalling during female gametogenesis | NOVA. The University of Newcastle's Digital Repository.

4. Bhattacharya P, Keating AF. Impact of environmental exposures on ovarian function and role of xenobiotic metabolism during ovotoxicity. *Toxicol Appl Pharmacol.* 2012;261(3):227–235.

5. Buffenstein R, Edrey YH, Yang T, Mele J. The oxidative stress theory of aging: embattled or invincible? Insights from non-traditional model organisms. *Age.* 2008;30(2–3):99–109.

6. Agarwal A, Gupta S, Sharma RK. Role of oxidative stress in female reproduction. *Reprod Biol Endocrinol.* 2005;3(28):1–21.

7. Benkhalifa M, Ferreira YJ, Chahine H, et al. Mitochondria: participation to infertility as source of energy and cause of senescence. *Int J Biochem Cell Biol.* 2014;55:60–64.

8. Ishii T, Miyazawa M, Takanashi Y, et al. Genetically induced oxidative stress in mice causes thrombocytosis, splenomegaly and placental angiodysplasia that leads to recurrent abortion. *Redox Biol.* 2014;2:679–685.

9. Pandey AN, Tripathi A, Premkumar KV, Shrivastav TG, Chaube SK. Reactive oxygen and nitrogen species during meiotic resumption from diplotene arrest in mammalian oocytes. *J Cell Biochem.* 2010;111(3):521–528. https://doi.org/10.1002/jcb.22736.

10. Tatemoto H, Sakurai N, Muto N. Protection of porcine oocytes against apoptotic cell death caused by oxidative stress during in vitro maturation: role of cumulus cells. *Biol Reprod.* 2000;63(3):805–810.

11. Shkolnik K, Tadmor A, Ben-Dor S, Nevo N, Galiani D, Dekel N. Reactive oxygen species are indispensable in ovulation. *Proc Natl Acad Sci USA.* 2011;108(4):1462–1467. https://doi.org/10.1073/pnas.1017213108.

12. Eichenlaub-Ritter U. Oocyte ageing and its cellular basis. *Int J Dev Biol.* 2012;56(10–12):841–852.

13. Boots C, Stephenson MD. Does obesity increase the risk of miscarriage in spontaneous conception: a systematic review. *Semin Reprod Med.* 2011;29(6):507–513. https://doi.org/10.1055/s-0031-1293204.

14. Bondia-Pons I, Ryan L, Martinez JA. Oxidative stress and inflammation interactions in human obesity. *J Physiol Biochem.* 2012;68(4):701–711. https://doi.org/10.1007/s13105-012-0154-2.

15. An Y, Wang Z, Ji H, Zhang Y, Wu K. Pituitary-adrenal and sympathetic nervous system responses to psychiatric disorders in women undergoing in vitro fertilization treatment. *Fertil Steril.* 2011;96(2):404–408.

16. Chiurchiù V, Orlacchio A, Maccarrone M. Is modulation of oxidative stress an answer? The state of the art of redox therapeutic actions in neurodegenerative diseases. *Oxid Med Cell Longev.* 2016;2016, 7909380.

17. Jesberger JA, Richardson JS. Oxygen free radicals and brain dysfunction. *Int J Neurosci.* 1991;57(1–2):1–17.

18. Alam F, Khan TA, Amjad S, Rehman R. Association of oxidative stress with female infertility—a case control study. *J Pak Med Assoc.* 2019;69(5):627–631.

19. Appasamy M, Jauniaux E, Serhal P, Al-Qahtani A, Groome NP, Muttukrishna S. Evaluation of the relationship between follicular fluid oxidative stress, ovarian hormones, and response to gonadotropin stimulation. *Fertil Steril.* 2008;89(4):912–921.

20. Rehman R, Jawaid S, Gul H, Khan R. Impact of peak estradiol levels on reproductive outcome of intracytoplasmic sperm injection. *Pak J Med Sci.* 2014;30(5):986.

21. Shanmugham D, Vidhyalakshmi R, Shivamurthy H. The effect of baseline serum luteinizing hormone levels on follicular development, ovulation, conception and pregnancy

outcome in infertile patients with polycystic ovarian syndrome. *Int J Reprod Contracept Obstet Gynecol.* 2017;7(1):318–322.

22. Merksamer PI, Liu Y, He W, Hirschey MD, Chen D, Verdin E. The sirtuins, oxidative stress and aging: an emerging link. *Aging (Albany NY).* 2013;5(3):144–150. https://doi.org/10.18632/aging.100544.
23. Morris BJ. Seven sirtuins for seven deadly diseases of aging. *Free Radic Biol Med.* 2013;56:133–171. https://doi.org/10.1016/j.freeradbiomed.2012.10.525.
24. North BJ, Verdin E. Sirtuins: Sir2-related NAD-dependent protein deacetylases. *Genome Biol.* 2004;5(5):224.
25. Brunet A, Sweeney LB, Sturgill JF, et al. Stress-dependent regulation of FOXO transcription factors by the SIRT1 deacetylase. *Science.* 2004;303(5666):2011–2015. https://doi.org/10.1126/science.1094637.
26. Rodgers JT, Lerin C, Haas W, Gygi SP, Spiegelman BM, Puigserver P. Nutrient control of glucose homeostasis through a complex of PGC-1alpha and SIRT1. *Nature.* 2005;434(7029):113–118. https://doi.org/10.1038/nature03354.
27. St-Pierre J, Drori S, Uldry M, et al. Suppression of reactive oxygen species and neurodegeneration by the PGC-1 transcriptional coactivators. *Cell.* 2006;127(2):397–408. https://doi.org/10.1016/j.cell.2006.09.024.
28. Pillarisetti S. A review of Sirt1 and Sirt1 modulators in cardiovascular and metabolic diseases. *Recent Pat Cardiovasc Drug Discov.* 2008;3(3):156–164.
29. Coussens M, Maresh JG, Yanagimachi R, Maeda G, Allsopp R. Sirt1 deficiency attenuates spermatogenesis and germ cell function. *PLoS One.* 2008;3(2):e1571. https://doi.org/10.1371/journal.pone.0001571.
30. Bordone L, Cohen D, Robinson A, et al. SIRT1 transgenic mice show phenotypes resembling calorie restriction. *Aging Cell.* 2007;6(6):759–767. https://doi.org/10.1111/j.1474-9726.2007.00335.x.
31. Moynihan KA, Grimm AA, Plueger MM, et al. Increased dosage of mammalian Sir2 in pancreatic β cells enhances glucose-stimulated insulin secretion in mice. *Cell Metab.* 2005;2(2):105–117.
32. Picard F, Kurtev M, Chung N, et al. Sirt1 promotes fat mobilization in white adipocytes by repressing PPAR-gamma. *Nature.* 2004;429(6993):771–776. https://doi.org/10.1038/nature02583.
33. Tao X, Zhang X, Ge SQ, Zhang EH, Zhang B. Expression of SIRT1 in the ovaries of rats with polycystic ovary syndrome before and after therapeutic intervention with exenatide. *Int J Clin Exp Pathol.* 2015;8(7):8276–8283.
34. Rehman R, Abidi SH, Alam F. Metformin, oxidative stress and infertility: a way forward. *Front Physiol.* 2018;9:1722.
35. Hukshorn CJ, Lindeman JHN, Toet KH, et al. Leptin and the proinflammatory state associated with human obesity. *J Clin Endocrinol Metabol.* 2004;89(4):1773–1778.
36. Tatone C, Di Emidio G, Vitti M, et al. Sirtuin functions in female fertility: possible role in oxidative stress and aging. *Oxid Med Cell Longev.* 2015;2015. https://doi.org/10.1155/2015/659687.
37. Tatone C, Di Emidio G, Barbonetti A, et al. Sirtuins in gamete biology and reproductive physiology: emerging roles and therapeutic potential in female and male infertility. *Hum Reprod Update.* 2018;24(3):267–289. https://doi.org/10.1093/humupd/dmy003.
38. Liu Y, He XQ, Huang X, et al. Resveratrol protects mouse oocytes from methylglyoxal-induced oxidative damage. *PLoS One.* 2013;8(10):e77960. https://doi.org/10.1371/journal.pone.0077960.

39. Ortega I, Duleba AJ. Ovarian actions of resveratrol. *Ann NY Acad Sci.* 2015;1348(1):86–96. https://doi.org/10.1111/nyas.12875.
40. Hussain SP, Amstad P, He P, et al. p53-induced up-regulation of MnSOD and GPX but not catalase increases oxidative stress and apoptosis. *Cancer Res.* 2004;64(7):2350–2356.
41. Zhao Y, Chaiswing L, Velez JM, et al. p53 translocation to mitochondria precedes its nuclear translocation and targets mitochondrial oxidative defense protein-manganese superoxide dismutase. *Cancer Res.* 2005;65(9):3745–3750.
42. Liu J, Liu M, Ye X, et al. Delay in oocyte aging in mice by the antioxidant N-acetyl-L-cysteine (NAC). *Hum Reprod.* 2012;27(5):1411–1420.
43. Solomon JM, Pasupuleti R, Xu L, et al. Inhibition of SIRT1 catalytic activity increases p53 acetylation but does not alter cell survival following DNA damage. *Mol Cell Biol.* 2006;26(1):28–38.
44. Ozden O, Park S-H, Kim H-S, et al. Acetylation of MnSOD directs enzymatic activity responding to cellular nutrient status or oxidative stress. *Aging (Albany NY).* 2011;3(2):102–107.
45. Peck B, Chen C-Y, Ho K-K, et al. SIRT inhibitors induce cell death and p53 acetylation through targeting both SIRT1 and SIRT2. *Mol Cancer Ther.* 2010;9(4):844–855.
46. Tatone C, Di Emidio G, Vento M, Ciriminna R, Artini PG. Cryopreservation and oxidative stress in reproductive cells. *Gynecol Endocrinol.* 2010;26(8):563–567. https://doi.org/10.3109/09513591003686395.
47. Kawamura Y, Uchijima Y, Horike N, ct al. Sirt3 protects in vitro-fertilized mouse preimplantation embryos against oxidative stress-induced p53-mediated developmental arrest. *J Clin Invest.* 2010;120(8):2817–2828. https://doi.org/10.1172/jci42020.
48. Morita Y, Wada-Hiraike O, Yano T, et al. Resveratrol promotes expression of SIRT1 and StAR in rat ovarian granulosa cells: an implicative role of SIRT1 in the ovary. *Reprod Biol Endocrinol.* 2012;10:14. https://doi.org/10.1186/1477-7827-10-14.
49. Canto C, Gerhart-Hines Z, Feige JN, et al. AMPK regulates energy expenditure by modulating NAD+ metabolism and SIRT1 activity. *Nature.* 2009;458(7241):1056–1060. https://doi.org/10.1038/nature07813.
50. Caton PW, Nayuni NK, Kieswich J, Khan NQ, Yaqoob MM, Corder R. Metformin suppresses hepatic gluconeogenesis through induction of SIRT1 and GCN5. *J Endocrinol.* 2010;205(1):97–106. https://doi.org/10.1677/joe-09-0345.
51. Behrman HR, Kodaman PH, Preston SL, Gao S. Oxidative stress and the ovary. *J Soc Gynecol Investig.* 2001;8(1 suppl. proceedings):S40–S42.
52. Bause AS, Haigis MC. SIRT3 regulation of mitochondrial oxidative stress. *Exp Gerontol.* 2013;48(7):634–639.
53. Perkins AV. Endogenous anti-oxidants in pregnancy and preeclampsia. *Aust NZ J Obstet Gynaecol.* 2006;46(2):77–83. https://doi.org/10.1111/j.1479-828X.2006.00532.x.
54. Lima AP, Moura MD, Rosa e Silva AA. Prolactin and cortisol levels in women with endometriosis. *Braz J Med Biol Res.* 2006;39(8):1121–1127.
55. Reverchon M, Cornuau M, Cloix L, et al. Visfatin is expressed in human granulosa cells: regulation by metformin through AMPK/SIRT1 pathways and its role in steroidogenesis. *Mol Hum Reprod.* 2013;19(5):313–326. https://doi.org/10.1093/molehr/gat002.
56. Gagarina V, Gabay O, Dvir-Ginzberg M, et al. SirT1 enhances survival of human osteoarthritic chondrocytes by repressing protein tyrosine phosphatase 1B and activating the insulin-like growth factor receptor pathway. *Arthritis Rheum.* 2010;62(5):1383–1392.
57. Chen S, Sun L, Gao H, Ren L, Liu N, Song G. Visfatin and oxidative stress influence endothelial progenitor cells in obese populations. *Endocr Res.* 2015;40(2):83–87.

58. Moreno-Vinasco L, Quijada H, Sammani S, et al. Nicotinamide phosphoribosyltransferase inhibitor is a novel therapeutic candidate in murine models of inflammatory lung injury. *Am J Respir Cell Mol Biol.* 2014;51(2):223–228.

59. Marseglia L, D'Angelo G, Manti M, et al. Visfatin: new marker of oxidative stress in preterm newborns. *Int J Immunopathol Pharmacol.* 2016;29(1):23–29.

60. Chu G, Yoshida K, Narahara S, et al. Alterations of circadian clockworks during differentiation and apoptosis of rat ovarian cells. *Chronobiol Int.* 2011;28(6):477–487. https://doi.org/10.3109/07420528.2011.589933.

61. Shen CJ, Tsai EM, Lee JN, Chen YL, Lee CH, Chan TF. The concentrations of visfatin in the follicular fluids of women undergoing controlled ovarian stimulation are correlated to the number of oocytes retrieved. *Fertil Steril.* 2010;93(6):1844–1850. https://doi.org/10.1016/j.fertnstert.2008.12.090.

62. Esplin MS, Fausett MB, Peltier MR, et al. The use of cDNA microarray to identify differentially expressed labor-associated genes within the human myometrium during labor. *Am J Obstet Gynecol.* 2005;193(2):404–413. https://doi.org/10.1016/j.ajog.2004.12.021.

63. Fasshauer M, Bluher M, Stumvoll M, Tonessen P, Faber R, Stepan H. Differential regulation of visfatin and adiponectin in pregnancies with normal and abnormal placental function. *Clin Endocrinol (Oxf).* 2007;66(3):434–439. https://doi.org/10.1111/j.1365-2265.2007.02751.x.

64. Garten A, Schuster S, Penke M, Gorski T, de Giorgis T, Kiess W. Physiological and pathophysiological roles of NAMPT and NAD metabolism. *Nat Rev Endocrinol.* 2015;11(9):535–546. https://doi.org/10.1038/nrendo.2015.117.

65. Reverchon M, Rame C, Bunel A, Chen W, Froment P, Dupont J. VISFATIN (NAMPT) improves in vitro IGF1-induced steroidogenesis and IGF1 receptor signaling through SIRT1 in bovine granulosa cells. *Biol Reprod.* 2016;94(3):54. https://doi.org/10.1095/biolreprod.115.134650.

66. Haider DG, Holzer G, Schaller G, et al. The adipokine visfatin is markedly elevated in obese children. *J Pediatr Gastroenterol Nutr.* 2006;43(4):548–549. https://doi.org/10.1097/01.mpg.0000235749.50820.b3.

67. Castrejón-Sosa M, Villalobos-Molina R, Guinzberg R, Piña E. Adrenaline (via α1B-adrenoceptors) and ethanol stimulate OH radical production in isolated rat hepatocytes. *Life Sci.* 2002;71(21):2469–2474.

68. Musalı N, Özmen B, Şükür YE, et al. Follicular fluid norepinephrine and dopamine concentrations are higher in polycystic ovary syndrome. *Gynecol Endocrinol.* 2016;32(6):460–463.

69. Abate NI, Mansour YH, Tuncel M, et al. Overweight and sympathetic overactivity in black Americans. *Hypertension.* 2001;38(3):379–383.

Assisted reproductive techniques

12

Sofia Amjad[a] and Rehana Rehman[b]

[a]*Department of Physiology, Ziauddin University, Karachi, Pakistan,* [b]*Department of Biological & Biomedical Sciences, Aga Khan University, Karachi, Pakistan*

Chapter outline

Introduction

"Assisted reproduction" is the support provided to address infertility issues. It refers to all methods that assist infertile couples to achieve pregnancy and give birth to their own babies.[1] Infertility rate in Pakistan is documented to be 21.9%, and the success rate is only 25% even after introduction of procedures like intracytoplasmic sperm injection (ICSI).[1] "Assisted reproductive techniques (ARTs)" are procedures that represent an amalgamation of development in physiology, endocrinology, pharmacology, diagnostic technology, and clinical care of infertile couples. These techniques are intended to overcome natural barriers in fertilization and include in vitro fertilization (IVF) of human gametes and embryo replacement into the uterine cavity with the goal of achieving pregnancy.[2]

Need of assisted reproductive technology

Since the first successful term birth with the help of ART procedure,[3] continued technological advancements have been made to refine ARTs for improved outcomes. The need for ARTs is correspondingly increasing with increasing awareness,

Subfertility. https://doi.org/10.1016/B978-0-323-75945-8.00012-8

advancement of new techniques, increase in the number and accessibility to fertility clinics, enthusiasm, and affordability of the couples to pursue treatments.[4]

Physiology of reproduction

During the process of reproduction, the male yields millions of gametes or spermatozoa, while the female yields a single female gamete or oocyte. In gametogenesis, haploid gametes are formed by meiosis of diploid progenitor cells that can fuse at the time of fertilization to produce a new, totally exclusive diploid organism. The homologous genetic recombination in prophase of meiosis I generates genetic diversity. This random combination of genetic material produces a variety of traits in the members of the species.[5]

The ejaculation of sperms into the female reproductive tract enables the process of fertilization. While passing through the female reproductive tract, the process of capacitation occurs in sperms with the removal of cholesterol from the membranes along with calcium influx, thus making the plasma membrane less stable.[6,7] In addition to this, the hyperactivated sperm motility and hyaluronidase secretion helps the sperm to penetrate the cumulus extracellular matrix for reaching the zona pellucida, where the capacitated sperm initiates acrosome reaction by binding of zona protein ZP3 with a sperm protein 1,4-galactosidase.[8] This reaction releases hydrolytic enzymes, including proacrosin, which are activated to acrosin. Acrosin along with the flagellar beating of sperm is important in digesting zona pellucida and penetration of sperm into the oocyte plasma membrane.[9] Then, the plasma membranes of sperm and oocyte fuse, by the interaction of sperm protein; Izumo1, and its cognate receptor, Juno, on the oolemma.[10] Ultimately, sperm nucleus moves into the egg cytoplasm and chromatids of sperm and oocyte condensate to form pronuclei, thus completing meiosis. Polyspermy is blocked by certain changes that include shedding of Juno receptors from the oolemma, oocyte membrane depolarization, and cortical granule secretion.[11]

Diploid zygote is formed by the combination and intermingling of the maternal and paternal chromosomes at syngamy, following the breakdown of pronuclear membranes.[5] After the first cleavage division, two-cell embryo is formed 28h after insemination, and the embryo undergoes several cleavage divisions forming a four-cell embryo at 44h and an eight-cell embryo at 68h. Beyond this eight-cell stage, embryo undergoes cell differentiation and enters the uterine cavity late on day 3 after fertilization.[12,13] The embryo reaches the blastocyst stage in 5–6days of fertilization, and after hatching from the zona pellucida, syncytial trophoblastic cells interact directly with the uterine epithelium through the stages of apposition, stable adhesion, and invasion.[14]

Factors affecting successful outcome of ARTs

The physiognomies and lifestyles of the individual undergoing that treatment have an indirect effect on the successful outcome of every procedure. Factors in both partners influence the success of an ART, though some elements have a more significant effect than others.

Maternal age: Female's age is an important factor to determine the successful outcome of the procedure. The comparative decrease in fertility of women in their late 30s has been reported to be half than the women in early 20s.[15] With a delay in the referral of females to infertility clinics, increased maternal age may contribute to a reduction in maturity and fertilization of oocytes.[1,16] Increasing age causes a diminution in the reproduction potential of women due to a decrease in the number of follicles, retrieved oocytes, and number of embryos.[17] It is reported that the higher follicle-stimulating hormone (FSH) levels in older patients are responsible for lower implantation rate.[18] Regarding all infertility treatment procedures, chances of success are diminished with age and a corresponding live birth rate is also decreased by 2% for each year with an increase in female age. The live birth rate per IVF cycle is about 26%–40% in females under the age of 35 years and decreases to about 6% above 40 years of age.[19]

Ovarian reserve: The ovarian reserve is mainly tested by follicle stimulating hormone (FSH), estradiol, anti-Müllerian hormone (AMH), and an ovarian antral follicle count (AFC). FSH is routinely done in clinical practice since it can also predict the response to ovarian stimulation.

Body mass index (BMI): Decline in natural fertility has been reported to be associated with obesity (BMI: $25.8–30.8 \, kg/m^2$). This can be due to either disturbed hypothalamic–pituitary–ovarian axis or ovulatory dysfunction induced by increased BMI. The rate of infertility in obese women is expected to increase by 4% per kg/m^2 rise in BMI.[15] The success of fertility treatments in obese individuals decreases to half when compared with normal weight individuals. Lower pregnancy rates and spontaneous abortion have also been reported in obese women after IVF or ICSI.[20]

Obesity in men (BMI $\geq 35 \, kg/m^2$) causes abnormalities in sexual function and sperm count with an increase in DNA fragmentation index. Possible mechanisms for fertility delay include rise in testicular temperature due to fat deposition, hyperinsulinemia, and affected hypothalamo-pituitary axis due to increased estrogen.[21]

Smoking and alcohol: Maternal and paternal smoking and alcohol consumption habits significantly influence the success of IVF. Female alcohol consumption was found to be associated with 13% decrease in the number of eggs aspirated, if alcohol was consumed 1 year prior to IVF or gamete intrafallopian transfer (GIFT) attempt. One-month prior use increases the risk of not achieving pregnancy by 2.86 times, and 1 week before the procedure, it increases the risk of miscarriage by 2.21 times.[15] Regarding alcohol consumption in men, it is documented that additional drink per day increases the risk of not achieving a live birth by 2.28–8.32 times; this also holds true for beer. The risk of miscarriage is increased by 2.70–38.04 times for men who drank 1 month before and during IVF and GIFT.[16] Smoking in both females and males affects success of ARTs, but caffeine consumption has no effect on natural fertility rates. Smoking in males is found to increase the risk of pregnancy loss, while female smoking causes an adverse effect on ovarian reserve.[22] The decrease in IVF success caused by lifestyle factors and poor nutritional habits is thought to be due to chronic oxidative stress.

Healthy lifestyles during the periconceptional period is a window of opportunity to attain successful ART outcomes. Therefore, by modifying behaviors, short-term reproductive health as well as general health can be improved.[15,23]

Types of assisted reproductive technology

ARTs comprise a number of procedures including intrauterine insemination (IUI), in vitro fertilization and embryo transfer (IVF-ET), GIFT, ZIFT, and ICSI.[24] The sequential approaches in assisted reproductive clinics are chosen from one of the following:

1. **Intrauterine insemination (IUI):** It is a type of ART in which the sperms are placed in the uterine cavity at the time of ovulation. It is a treatment of choice in a natural cycle with or without ovarian stimulation by oral antiestrogens or gonadotropins. The success of IUI and timed intercourse (TI) is almost the same.[25]
2. **In vitro fertilization and embryo transfer (IVF-ET):** In IVF, one or more fertilized eggs (embryos) are inserted to nurture in the uterine cavity. Excess embryos are kept for future frozen embryo transfer cycles (FET). Initially, IVF was recommended only for problems in fallopian tubes. Nowadays, it is extended to include other causes like endometriosis, male factor, or unexplained infertility. IVF is the most commonly used technique and the mainstay of ART, since ET can be achieved in the same cycle, or cryopreserved embryos could be transferred in a subsequent cycle (Table 12.1).[26]
3. **Gamete intrafallopian transfer (GIFT):** It is not widely used nowadays, and technique of this is much of the same as IVF. In this procedure, eggs are collected the same way as in IVF, but are transferred laparoscopically along with the motile sperm to the fallopian tube for in vivo fertilization.[25,27] It is recommended for cases, where infertility is due to an unexplained male factor.
4. **Zygote intrafallopian transfer (ZIFT):** In this procedure, embryo is developed in vitro, but is transferred laparoscopically to the fallopian tube. It is specifically used in situations, where transcervical gamete transfer is not possible.[28] However, with the latest advancements in "in vitro" conditions supporting normal fertilization and preimplantation embryo development, GIFT and ZIFT are no longer in use.[5]
5. **Intracytoplasmic sperm injection (ICSI):** It is a technique by which a morphologically normal and motile single spermatozoon is injected directly into the ooplasm through the process of micromanipulation. Sperm is selected on the basis of its motility and morphology for ICSI.

Assisted reproductive technology treatment cycle

An ART treatment cycle is a process through which a woman undergoes multiple steps of this procedure, including pituitary downregulation, controlled ovarian stimulation, ovulation induction, oocyte and sperm retrieval, fertilization, ET, and luteal

Table 12.1 Comparison of IVF and other assisted procedures.

IVF (in vitro fertilization)	GIFT (gamete intrafallopian transfer)	ZIFT (zygote intrafallopian transfer)
• IVF can be done in many causes of male and female infertility	• Used in male factor fertility problem and unexplained fertility problem where woman has normal tubes	• Used where transcervical gamete transfer is not possible
• The eggs and sperms are fertilized outside the womb	• The egg is fertilized in the tube	• Fertilization is done in a laboratory outside the body
• The zygote is transferred to the woman's uterus	• The gametes (egg and sperm) are transferred to the woman's fallopian tubes and not the uterus	• The gametes are fertilized in the laboratory, and the fertilized egg is transferred to the tube rather than the uterus
• One or more embryos are drawn into a transfer catheter and placed in the uterus	• Laparoscopy is mandatory to transfer the sperm and egg to the tubes	• Laparoscopy is mandatory to transfer the zygote to the tubes
• Fertilization confirmed when embryos are transferred	• Fertilization cannot be confirmed as with IVF	• Fertilization cannot be confirmed as with IVF
• Most commonly used ART method	• Comprises less than 1% of ART procedures	• Comprises less than 1% of ART procedures

support. The appropriate management of these steps is crucial for a good reproductive outcome of ART.[4]

Pre-assisted reproductive technology (pre-ART) strategies

Pre-ART strategies are meant to start before ART cycle in order to improve the reproductive outcome of treatment. These strategies include the following:

Pre-ART hormonal treatment: It is for the development of follicle and endometrium recommended as per National Institute for Health and Care Excellence (NICE) guidelines.[4,29] It has been reported that the chances of pregnancy increase fourfolds when a gonadotropin-releasing hormone (GnRH) agonist is used for a period of 3–6months, especially in women with endometriosis-associated infertility.[30]

Pre-ART surgical and other interventions: Other intervention strategies recommend the use of antioxidants, vasodilators, metformin, and surgical procedures.

Steps of ART cycle (Fig. 12.1)

Pituitary downregulation: This is done temporarily to suppress the pituitary gland's release of gonadotropins and premature ovulation from early exposure to luteinizing

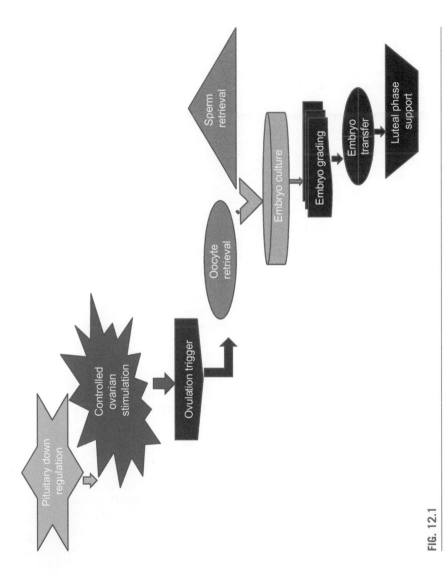

FIG. 12.1

Flowchart of steps of in vitro fertilization–embryo transfer (IVF-ET).

hormone (LH). This pituitary downregulation ensures that the oocytes are available for retrieval prior to insemination in the laboratory. The downregulation protocols are selected on the basis of maternal age, ovarian reserve, BMI, past history (medical, endocrine, and fertility), preference of the clinician or center, and the patient's previous outcome and anticipated ovarian response.[4,15]

Downregulation is achieved by using either GnRH agonists or antagonist.[31] In the long GnRH agonist (GnRH-a) treatment cycle, exogenous gonadotropins are administered to prevent early LH surge, which increases the number of retrieved oocytes. However, GnRH-a may lead to ovarian hyperstimulation syndrome (OHSS) or other side effects.[32] In GnRH antagonist (GnRH-ant) protocols, GnRH receptors are competitively blocked and gonadotropin release is suppressed. This protocol is more convenient as it is a short-term treatment for ovarian stimulation with fewer complications.[33] It has been observed that a single use of long-acting GnRH-ant during the luteal phase is more beneficial, as it combines the effects of both antagonist and agonist protocols.[33] In patients with normal or high ovarian reserve, GnRH-ant protocol reduces the incidence of OHSS considerably; however, the pregnancy rate and live birth rate are the same as with GnRH-a long protocol.[32] The antagonist protocol in high responders eliminates the need for complete cryopreservation of embryos.[34] In women with a predicted poor ovarian response, evidence suggests that a shorter course of the GnRH-ant protocol is required.[35]

Controlled ovarian stimulation (COS): In a normal menstrual cycle, almost 10–20 ovarian antral follicles start developing in each ovary, of which only one grows dominantly over the others, until ovulation occurs.[18] During COS, medications are used to stimulate the growth of multiple mature eggs for surgical retrieval, prior to IVF. Stimulation with gonadotropins containing FSH produces multifollicular development instead of mono-ovulation so that more than one oocyte can be retrieved.[4]

Plan to initiate COS is important in an IVF cycle. The response is monitored by using two-dimensional transvaginal ultrasound scans to measure the development of ovarian follicles. Blood samples are also drawn to gauge the level of hormones in response to COS medications. Normally, estrogen levels increase with the development of follicles, while progesterone levels drop until after ovulation. The stimulation dose and response to the medication are monitored to assess the final maturation of follicles for retrieval. In case of underresponse and hyperresponse, it also enables the clinician to make a decision to cancel ART cycle.[36,37]

Ovulation trigger: Blood tests and ultrasound scans enable the physician to determine whether the follicles are ready for egg retrieval. By the end of the stimulation phase (8–14 days of treatment), a hormone is given to cause the midcycle LH surge so that eggs could be retrieved before ovulation occurs. Urinary human chorionic gonadotropin, recombinant human chorionic gonadotropin (rhCG), and recombinant luteinizing hormone (rLH) have been used to trigger final oocyte maturation. The human chorionic gonadotropin (hCG) injection is given 34–36 hours before ovulation for ultimate follicular maturation and resumption of meiosis, thus contributing to ovulation, follicular luteinization and formation of corpus luteum. Live births, ongoing pregnancy rates, and rates of OHSS are not affected by the type of recombinant drugs. Urinary hCG is the preferred choice for ovulation trigger in ART cycles because it is less expensive, safe, and equally effective as rhCG and rLH.[38] In addition to this, the risk of OHSS is reduced by giving a small dose of hCG after a GnRH-a trigger, whereas in a low-risk group, a second dose of hCG is also given.[39]

Oocyte retrieval: After the ovulation trigger, mature oocytes are retrieved from the ovaries using the gold standard, ultrasound-guided transvaginal probe used in IVF.[40] To decrease the chance of spontaneous ovulation, retrieval is usually performed 36 hours after the preovulatory trigger to get the most of mature oocytes.[5] In patients with severe obesity, large-sized uterine fibroids, Müllerian anomalies, or prior oophoropexy, the ovaries are inaccessible and oocyte retrieval by transvaginal route is not possible. In such cases, transabdominal ultrasound or laparoscopic oocyte retrieval is done under sedation and analgesia.[41]

Follicular fluid with retrieved oocyte is placed in test tubes containing N-2-hydroxyethylpiperazine-N'-2-ethanesulfonic acid (HEPES)-buffered media so that isolation of the cumulus oophorus complexes can be done in the embryology laboratory to assess their maturity and quality. The assessment of nuclear and cytoplasmic maturation, by the absence of germinal vesical and presence of the first polar body, is done to confirm the maturation of an oocyte and early embryonic development. Mature eggs are placed in the incubator for about 4 h until insemination is done.[5]

Sperm retrieval: Sperm sample for ART is obtained by masturbation without lubricants after 2–5 days of abstinence. In obstructive azoospermia or ejaculatory failure, the sperm is taken directly from the testes using surgical techniques like percutaneous epididymal sperm aspiration, testicular sperm aspiration, and microscopic epididymal sperm aspiration. In nonobstructive azoospermia, microscopic testicular sperm extraction or open testicular biopsies are required.[42]

The success of sperm retrieval relays on the etiology of infertility whether azoospermia is obstructive or nonobstructive and the type of procedure involved to retrieve it. It has been reported that in obstructive azoospermia, the sperm retrieval success rate is 78%–100% as compared to 34%–92% in nonobstructive azoospermia. It has also been observed that the reproductive outcome is poor if sperm is obtained from nonobstructive azoospermia.[29] The sperm sample is processed and placed in the incubator until insemination or ICSI for fertilization. Insemination procedure is selected on the basis of sperm count and morphology: IVF is chosen for patients with high sperm count and normal sperm morphology, whereas ICSI is chosen for patients with poor sperm quality, antisperm antibodies, and in patients with the previous failure of IVF cycle.[15]

Embryo culture: After insemination or ICSI, the oocytes are kept in the incubator for 18 h, whereby fertilization is identified by the presence of two pronuclei in the oocytes. The fertilized oocytes are placed in the incubator for another day. Then from day 2 till day 6, embryo is scored according to the number of blastomeres present in it: day 2 embryos have four blastomeres, day 3 embryos have eight blastomeres, day 4 embryos have compacted stage, while day 5 and day 6 embryos have blastocyst stage.[18]

Embryo grading: Different techniques are used to evaluate the quality of an embryo to identify the one that is most likely to get implanted leading to successful live birth. Invasive methods used for embryo evaluation include preimplantation genetic screening and metabolomics, while noninvasive method is static morphologic grading.[4,5] Morphological grading, which remains the first line of approach for grading of the embryos, is done at definite intervals during the incubation period according to blastomere number, blastomere size, and fragmentation to determine the cleavage stage of the embryo. Other features to be noted include multinucleated blastomeres, vacuolation, granularity, and zona defects.[43]

Embryo transfer: After the embryo culture, one or two of the resultant embryos in the cleavage phase (days 2/3) or blastocyst phase (days 5/6) are transferred into the midfundal portion of the uterus through a catheter.[5] A higher clinical pregnancy rate and live birth rate have been reported with the blastocyst stage transfer.[44]

Luteal phase support: After the COS and oocyte retrieval, a number of corpora lutea in the ovaries are formed that produce large amounts of steroids. This increase in steroids decreases the synthesis of LH by a negative feedback mechanism and premature luteolysis, which can lead to pregnancy loss.[45] Therefore, after oocyte pickup, luteal phase support is given by direct or indirect replacement of progesterone (with or without estrogen) to correct LH deficiency.[29]

Embryo cryopreservation: In some circumstances, oocytes may be collected and frozen for later transfer. This is a type of IVF cycle that is divided into two phases: COS and deferred ET.[46] This approach helps in the optimization of embryo-endometrial synchrony, prevents OHSS, and provides time for preimplantation genetic testing.[47]

Pregnancy test: The implantation of the embryo(s) is confirmed by testing urinary or serum beta-hCG around 2 weeks after the oocyte retrieval.

Early pregnancy scan: Ultrasound scan is done at 7 weeks of gestation once the pregnancy test is positive. An early scan is recommended in women with a previous history of ectopic pregnancy or recurrent miscarriage, or with symptoms of bleeding or pain.[4]

An IVF cycle can be stopped at any point, if the woman shows no response to treatment or presents with any risk, especially OHSS.

Potential risks associated with the steps of ART cycle

There are potential medical and surgical risks that may be associated with each step of the ART procedure. These have been listed in Table 12.2.

Table 12.2 Potential risks associated with ART cycle.

1	Controlled ovarian stimulation (COS)	A risk of hyperstimulation OHSS in which the ovaries become swollen and painful. Mild and moderate OHSS requires outpatient management. Rarely, severe OHSS needs hospitalization
2	Use of fertility medication	The role of fertility drugs with increased risk of ovarian cancer is not established; however, frequent follow-ups are recommended for all women
3	Retrieval of eggs	• Include risk of anesthesia, slight risk of bleeding while removing eggs • Infection • If the physician uses laparoscopy or ultrasound to guide the needle, risk of damage to the bowel, bladder, or a blood vessel
4	Chance of multiple pregnancies	With the transfer of more than one embryo chance exists and multiple pregnancies have their own problems like preterm birth and need special care
5	Miscarriage	Chances vary with age and are lesser in women younger than 35 years of age
6	Ectopic pregnancy	Minimal chance of ectopic pregnancy with IVF
7	Birth defects	Research is ongoing to establish a relation
8	Psychological stress	Anxiety and depression, especially if ART fails

References

1. Rehman R, Mahmood H, Syed F, Syed H, Gul H. Intracytoplasmic sperm injection and advanced maternal age: success or treatment failure. *Pak J Pharm Sci.* 2019;32(4):1495.
2. Sunderam S, Kissin DM, Zhang Y, et al. Assisted reproductive technology surveillance—United States, 2016. *MMWR Surveill Summ.* 2019;68(4):1–23.
3. Steptoe PC, Edwards RG. Birth after reimplantation of a human embryo. *Lancet.* 1978;2(8085):366.
4. Bhandari HM, Choudhary MK, Stewart JA. An overview of assisted reproductive technology procedures. *Obstet Gynaecol.* 2018;20(3):167–176.
5. Barbieri RL, Strauss JF. *Yen & Jaffe's Reproductive Endocrinology: Physiology, Pathophysiology, and Clinical Management.* Elsevier Saunders; 2014.
6. De Jonge C. Biological basis for human capacitation—revisited. *Hum Reprod Update.* 2017;23(3):289–299.
7. Gadella B, Boerke A. An update on post-ejaculatory remodeling of the sperm surface before mammalian fertilization. *Theriogenology.* 2016;85(1):113–124.
8. Reid AT, Redgrove K, Aitken RJ, Nixon B. Cellular mechanisms regulating sperm–zona pellucida interaction. *Asian J Androl.* 2011;13(1):88.
9. Georgadaki K, Khoury N, Spandidos DA, Zoumpourlis V. The molecular basis of fertilization. *Int J Mol Med.* 2016;38(4):979–986.
10. Bianchi E, Doe B, Goulding D, Wright GJ. Juno is the egg Izumo receptor and is essential for mammalian fertilization. *Nature.* 2014;508(7497):483.

11. Aston KI, Punj V, Liu L, Carrell DT. Genome-wide sperm deoxyribonucleic acid methylation is altered in some men with abnormal chromatin packaging or poor in vitro fertilization embryogenesis. *Fertil Steril.* 2012;97(2):285–292. e284.

12. Braude P, Bolton V, Moore S. Human gene expression first occurs between the four- and eight-cell stages of preimplantation development. *Nature.* 1988;332(6163):459–461.

13. Croxatto H, Ortiz M, Diaz S, Hess R, Balmaceda J, Croxatto H-D. Studies on the duration of egg transport by the human oviduct: II. Ovum location at various intervals following luteinizing hormone peak. *Am J Obstet Gynecol.* 1978;132(6):629–634.

14. Lindenberg S, Hyttel P, Lenz S, Holmes PV. Ultrastructure of the early human implantation in vitro. *Hum Reprod.* 1986;1(8):533–538.

15. Kovacs G. *The Subfertility Handbook: A Clinician's Guide.* Cambridge University Press; 2010.

16. Ye J, Luo D, Xu X, et al. Metformin improves fertility in obese males by alleviating oxidative stress-induced blood-testis barrier damage. *Oxid Med Cell Longev.* 2019;2019, 9151067.

17. Karimzadeh MA, Ghandi S, Tabibnejad N. Age as a predictor of assisted reproductive techniques outcome. *Pak J Med Sci.* 2008;24(3):378.

18. Rehman R, Irfan T, Jawed S, Hussain M, Ali R. Embryo quality in intracytoplasmic sperm injection: a quasi experimental design in Pakistan. J Pak Med Assoc 2018;68(10):1451–1455.

19. Wright VC, Schieve LA, Reynolds MA, Jeng G. Assisted reproductive technology surveillance—United States, 2002. *MMWR Surveill Summ.* 2005;54(2):1–24.

20. Li X-L, Huang R, Fang C, Wang Y-F, Liang X-Y. Logistic regression analysis of risk factors associated with spontaneous abortion after in vitro fertilization/intracytoplasmic sperm injection-embryo transfer in polycystic ovary syndrome patients. *Reprod Dev Med.* 2018;2(2):105.

21. Kahn BE, Brannigan RE. Obesity and male infertility. *Curr Opin Urol.* 2017;27(5):441–445.

22. Zitzmann M, Rolf C, Nordhoff V, et al. Male smokers have a decreased success rate for in vitro fertilization and intracytoplasmic sperm injection. *Fertil Steril.* 2003;79:1550–1554.

23. Oostingh EC, Hall J, Koster MP, Grace B, Jauniaux E, Steegers-Theunissen RP. The impact of maternal lifestyle factors on periconception outcomes: a systematic review of observational studies. *Reprod Biomed Online.* 2019;38(1):77–94.

24. Merchant R, Gandhi G, Allahbadia GN. In vitro fertilization/intracytoplasmic sperm injection for male infertility. *Indian J Urol.* 2011;27(1):121.

25. Veltman-Verhulst SM, Hughes E, Ayeleke RO, Cohlen BJ. Intra-uterine insemination for unexplained subfertility. *Cochrane Database Syst Rev.* 2016;2, CD001838.

26. Kamath MS, Bhattacharya S. Demographics of infertility and management of unexplained infertility. *Best Pract Res Clin Obstet Gynaecol.* 2012;26(6):729–738.

27. Wessels PH, Cronjé HS, Oosthuizen AP, Trümpelmann MD, Grobler S, Hamlett DK. Cost-effectiveness of gamete intrafallopian transfer in comparison with induction of ovulation with gonadotropins in the treatment of female infertility: a clinical trial. *Fertil Steril.* 1992;57(1):163–167.

28. Habana AE, Palter SF. Is tubal embryo transfer of any value? A meta-analysis and comparison with the Society for Assisted Reproductive Technology database. *Fertil Steril.* 2001;76(2):286–293.

29. National Institute for Health and Clinical Excellence: Guidance, National Collaborating Centre for Women's and Children's Health. *Fertility: Assessment and Treatment for People With Fertility Problems.* London: Royal College of Obstetricians and Gynaecologists; 2013.

30. Sallam HN, Garcia-Velasco JA, Dias S, Arici A, Abou-Setta AM. Long-term pituitary down-regulation before in vitro fertilization (IVF) for women with endometriosis. *Cochrane Database Syst Rev.* 2006;1, CD004635.

31. Vela G, Ruman J, Luna M, Sandler B, Copperman A. Profound pituitary suppression following oral contraceptive pretreatment in gonadotropin-releasing hormone antagonist cycles does not impact outcome: a retrospective cohort study. *JFIV Reprod Med Genet.* 2017;5(200):18–20.

32. Wang R, Lin S, Wang Y, Qian W, Zhou L. Comparisons of GnRH antagonist protocol versus GnRH agonist long protocol in patients with normal ovarian reserve: a systematic review and meta-analysis. *PLoS One.* 2017;12(4), e0175985.

33. Papanikolaou EG, Yarali H, Timotheou E, et al. A proof-of-concept clinical trial of a single luteal use of long-acting gonadotropin-releasing hormone antagonist degarelix in controlled ovarian stimulation for in vitro fertilization: long antagonist protocol. *Front Endocrinol.* 2018;9:25.

34. Nelson SM, Yates RW, Lyall H, et al. Anti-Müllerian hormone-based approach to controlled ovarian stimulation for assisted conception. *Hum Reprod.* 2009;24(4):867–875.

35. Xiao J, Chang S, Chen S. The effectiveness of gonadotropin-releasing hormone antagonist in poor ovarian responders undergoing in vitro fertilization: a systematic review and meta-analysis. *Fertil Steril.* 2013;100(6). 1594–1601.e1599.

36. Kwan I, Bhattacharya S, Kang A, Woolner A. Monitoring of stimulated cycles in assisted reproduction (IVF and ICSI). *Cochrane Database Syst Rev.* 2014;(8), CD005289.

37. Martins WP, Vieira C, Teixeira D, Barbosa M, Dassunção L, Nastri C. Ultrasound for monitoring controlled ovarian stimulation: a systematic review and meta-analysis of randomized controlled trials. *Ultrasound Obstet Gynecol.* 2014;43(1):25–33.

38. Youssef MA, Abou-Setta AM, Lam WS. Recombinant versus urinary human chorionic gonadotrophin for final oocyte maturation triggering in IVF and ICSI cycles. *Cochrane Database Syst Rev.* 2016;(4), CD003719.

39. Humaidan P, Polyzos N, Alsbjerg B, et al. GnRHa trigger and individualized luteal phase hCG support according to ovarian response to stimulation: two prospective randomized controlled multi-centre studies in IVF patients. *Hum Reprod.* 2013;28(9):2511–2521.

40. Leung AS, Dahan MH, Tan SL. *Techniques and Technology for Human Oocyte Collection.* Taylor & Francis; 2016.

41. Barton SE, Politch JA, Benson CB, Ginsburg ES, Gargiulo AR. Transabdominal follicular aspiration for oocyte retrieval in patients with ovaries inaccessible by transvaginal ultrasound. *Fertil Steril.* 2011;95(5):1773–1776.

42. Miyaoka R, Esteves SC. Sperm retrieval techniques. In: *Male Infertility.* Springer; 2020:621–635.

43. Cutting R, Morroll D, Roberts SA, et al. Elective single embryo transfer: guidelines for practice British Fertility Society and Association of Clinical Embryologists. *Hum Fertil.* 2008;11(3):131–146.

44. Gardner DK, Schoolcraft WB. Culture and transfer of human blastocysts. *Curr Opin Obstet Gynecol.* 1999;11(3):307–311.

45. van der Linden M, Buckingham K, Farquhar C, Kremer JA, Metwally M. Luteal phase support for assisted reproduction cycles. *Cochrane Database Syst Rev.* 2015;7, CD009154.

46. Devroey P, Polyzos NP, Blockeel C. An OHSS-Free Clinic by segmentation of IVF treatment. *Hum Reprod.* 2011;26(10):2593–2597.

47. Shapiro BS, Daneshmand ST, Garner FC, Aguirre M, Hudson C, Thomas S. Evidence of impaired endometrial receptivity after ovarian stimulation for in vitro fertilization: a prospective randomized trial comparing fresh and frozen–thawed embryo transfer in normal responders. *Fertil Steril.* 2011;96(2):344–348.

Way forward

13

Rehana Rehman

Department of Biological & Biomedical Sciences, Aga Khan University, Karachi, Pakistan

Chapter outline

Fertility awareness

In our society, fertility awareness (FA) is deficient, since cultural and religious factors increase the prevalence of misconceptions and myths. Core factors encompass low education, persistent health-related issues, scarcity of resources for well-being, nonexistence of a developed public health system, and inadequate coverage by insurance policies. Contributing factors include poor access to fertility options, scarce knowledge about risk factors for infertility, and health warnings of postponing childbirth (Fig. 13.1).

According to a study conducted in Pakistan, the reported prevalence of infertility is approximately 22% with 4% primary and 18% secondary infertility.[1] The cultural and religious perspective about assisted reproductive technologies is also unclear, resulting in reduced acceptability.[1]

Sufficient knowledge about infertility can urge young couples to seek timely medical care. We, therefore, recommend that infertile couples should be guided to approach the right person at the right time. Theinfertility clinics must have a list of relevant books and articles in local languages, audiovisuals, brochures, as well as the services of counselors who deals with fertility-related matters of individuals of different educational status. Additionally mass communication should play a very

Subfertility. https://doi.org/10.1016/B978-0-323-75945-8.00013-X

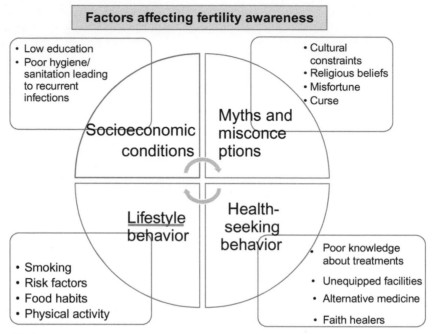

FIG. 13.1

Factors effecting fertility awareness.

effective role to address misconceptions, myths, and religious taboos through health shows and discussion forums with popular celebrities/health ambassadors. Support of religious authorities should also be obtained through sensitization meetings, so as to research and clarify any misconceptions at different forums portraying the correct Islamic views on treatment options such as IVF, for better acceptability.[1]

Role of healthcare professionals: First line of contact

In United Kingdom, Germany, and other developed countries, counseling of infertile couples and diagnostic evaluation come under the domain of primary care physicians. Counseling is offered at the time of first consultation and during the procedure by a person/specialist/psychologist who has a limited role in the management of the couple.[2] According to the American Society for Reproductive Medicine (ASRM), these counseling techniques offered on case-to-case basis will enable the couples to face physical and emotional challenges of infertility and its treatment.[3] Measures to improve general health through lifestyle modifications should also be included in this process. Comprehensive knowledge of the counselor and counseling skills can therefore decrease the perceived stress of subfertile couples and, therefore, improve treatment consequences.[4] Once counseled and diagnosed properly, the couple can be offered the first line of treatment, failing which immediate referral is planned.

Unfortunately, a majority of subfertility patients belong to developing countries, where negative consequences of childlessness are more as compared to developed countries.[5] Fertility awareness is minimal; cultural limitations, treatable recurrent infections, poor access to health facilities, and lack of appropriate counseling pose a serious threat to fertility. Access to newer technologies is rare, being costly and limited to big cities, making it unaffordable for a majority. Insignificant resources and low commitment of the government darken the scenario further. We postulate that the healthcare providers in primary care settings, being the first line of contact with the couple, can play a pivotal role to prevent infertility. Awareness and counseling sessions in the initial stages educate the patients about risk factors, which facilitate screening for and treating preventable causes, thus promoting patient compliance since "Beauty has no age; Fertility does."[5]

Counseling may be supported through print media (brochures) and where facilities exist, online modules and awareness workshops. If the couple does not conceive in a year's time, the healthcare professional should proceed with prompt referral to infertility specialist.

Fertility in primary healthcare settings: Challenges and solutions

Infertility treatment in low socioeconomic countries is a stand-alone. Knowing the status of education and prevention in developing countries, efforts are required at national level to develop administrative guidelines, to incorporate infertility into primary-level reproductive healthcare programs. For the successful inclusion of infertility diagnosis in these circumstances, it is necessary that the knowledge and skills of healthcare workers should be updated through ongoing, regular training programs. Sufficient facilities should also be made available for routine investigations, since early identification of cause and prompt treatment can minimize complications of procedures. While the diagnosis and treatment of infertility are comparatively expensive, it is recommended that more advanced, operational, secure, and cost-effective ART strategies should be proposed by public and private sectors.[6] A possible solution can be government's initiatives to pledge low-cost IVF programs, supplemented with funding from international agencies and other resources. Agencies from the private sectors should also be invited to join hands to address awareness issues and mass communication to improve the quality of care for subfertility.[7]

WHO recommendations and fertility counseling

To address fertility issues in the broader concept of medical, social, cultural, and religious dictums, it is a prerequisite that all activities are integrated at three levels, namely personal, interpersonal, and social.[1] World Health Organization (WHO) and Human Fertilization and Embryology Authority (HFEA) recommend that instead of individuals, couples seeking fertility treatment should be counseled.[8] Both partners should be approached together and counseled so that they accept one another's feelings and face challenges collectively. Where cultural constraints prevail, individual counseling may additionally be done to reduce stress[9] in infertile women. Counseling services and materials should be available, depending upon the educational status of couples/individuals and local circumstances/languages. Keeping in mind the diverse counseling needs of infertile couples, options of a number of suitable psychosocial provisions and counseling intermediations[10] come up. At personal level, steps to improve preventative behavior through awareness programs will help prevent the treatable. According to the recommendations of WHO, "*Public awareness of infertility and its causes should be increased to improve preventative behavior and to diminish the stigmatization and social exclusion of infertile men and women.*"[11] Research has found that being open about infertility and seeking support from outside can help both men and women cope better with emotional distress.[12] Social support comes from friends, family, and support groups, since they allow one to be better understood; to share feelings and emotions that could not have been shared anywhere else. A time and cost-efficient method of group counseling can be organized in the form of small groups to reduce social isolation, educate couples, discuss their problems, share experiences, convey information, teach and practice relaxation skills, and then identify couples for further psychological support.[13] Access to helpline maintains confidentiality in a two-way communication process and helps to remove misconceptions contributing to behavior change.[14]

Advanced counseling

Reproductive health and the field of subfertility can additionally benefit from the specialized services of a health coach, an individual who fills the gap between patient and doctor, to impart knowledge to the patient for improved attitude and practices of self-care. Once the diagnosis of infertility is established, couples should be counseled in detail on treatment choices available. For those who opt for IVF/ICSI, a detailed discussion is required on the nature of problem, chances, possibilities, and assistances of IVF in agreement with the current Human Fertilization and Embryology Authority (HFEA) code of practice.[2] To improve compliance, they should be informed about the length of intervention, that a complete cycle of IVF comprises of downregulation, ovarian stimulation, ovulation induction, embryo transfer, and cryopreservation of frozen embryo(s). Relaxation techniques including yoga meditation have been proved to reduce the perceived stress[15] supporting success after IVF or ICSI.[16]

Infertility clinic: First visit protocols

The first visit calls for a realistic, evidence-based protocol for the management of infertile couples rather than bombarding them with information overload.[17] A multidisciplinary approach is therefore required for a good clinical practice, following principles of care that the couple anticipates throughout treatment. This understanding may help infertility specialists to recognize and support couples who have a greater possibility of emotional distress, during various phases of interventions.[18] It includes the following.

History taking, examination, and routine investigations

History taking and examination of both partners individually and then collectively with focus on duration of infertility, number of previous ART treatment cycles, treatment protocols, results of fertilization and psychological adjustment throughout the cycle,[18] followed by routine investigations (Tables 13.1–13.6).

Counseling is required at each step of procedure to promote compliance.

Table 13.1 Infertility management protocol: history of female partner.

S. no.	History	Inclusions
1	Present history	• Elements of current problem, length of infertility in years, age, occupation
		• Associated conditions of vaginal/cervical discharge, hair growth, acne, breast change, hot flushes, change in dietary habits, symptoms of diabetes, hypertension, history of drugs, smoking, consumption of alcohol, and intake of caffeine
2	Menstrual history	• Onset of menarche, duration, and frequency of the cycle, relevant complaints
3	Obstetric history	• Previous conceptions (gravidity), parity, miscarriages
		• Induced abortion and its complications
4	Contraceptive history	• Type of contraceptives, duration of use
5	Sexual history	• Living together
		• Enough time for relation
		• Knowledge about timing of relation

		• Relevant complaints associated:
		  • Difficult coitus
		  • Pain during coitus

6	Past history	• Medical: rubella status, pelvic inflammatory diseases, tuberculosis
		• Surgical: removal of ovarian cysts, appendicectomy, open/laparoscopic laparotomy, previous cesarean section, cervical conization

7	Family history	• Especially important in cases of subfertility:
		  • PCOS and endometriosis, cousin marriages
		  • Diabetes mellitus, hypertension, twin's birth, breast cancer

Adopted from Kamel R: Management of the infertile couple: an evidence-based protocol, Reprod Biol Endocrinol 8(1):21, 2010. https://doi.org/10.1186/1477-7827-8-21.

Table 13.2 Infertility management protocol: history of male partner.

S. no.	History	Inclusions
1	Present history	• Age of male partner • Profession • Reports of previously conducted semen analysis • Breast enlargement • Associated conditions: symptoms of diabetes, hypertension, history of drugs, smoking, consumption of alcohol, and caffeine drinking
2	Sexual history	• Frequency, timing, erectile problem • Ejaculation dysfunction • Decrease of libido • Previous marital history, extramarital sexual activities
3	Medical history	• Mumps infection • Respiratory/gastrointestinal tuberculosis • Sexually transmitted diseases • Undescended testis

4	Contraceptive history	• Any method of contraception employed:
		  • Temporary (condom)
		  • Permanent (vasectomy)

5	Surgical history	• Appendectomy • Repair of inguinal hernia • Suspension surgeries of the urinary bladder neck
6	Family history	• Relevant medical and surgical histories

Adopted from Kamel R: Management of the infertile couple: an evidence-based protocol, Reprod Biol Endocrinol 8(1):21, 2010. https://doi.org/10.1186/1477-7827-8-21.

Counseling on lifestyle modifications

- Smoking: If required, female smokers should be *referred to a smoking cessation program* since both active and passive smoking influence fertility. The impact of smoking on general health and sperm parameters should also be informed.[19]
- Folic acid supplementation and other "*natural therapies can be added if prescribed by the physician.*"
- Obesity: *Women with a body mass index (BMI)≥30* should be counseled *to reduce weight* to increase the response to infertility treatment and conception. *A healthy lifestyle with good eating habits and regular physical activity* should be emphasized. On the same note, *men with a BMI≥30* should be warned *to reduce weight* to improve fertility.[20–22]
- Women with *BMI < 19* should be advised *to increase body weight.*
- Frequency and timing of sexual intercourse: Couples should be educated about "*timed sexual intercourse*" to increase the chance of pregnancy.
- Men should be warned to *avoid tight underwear.*

Table 13.3 Infertility management protocol: general physical examination of female partner.

S. no.	Examination	Inclusions
1	General	• Estimation of blood pressure • Body height and weight (BMI) = ratio of weight (kilograms) with height (square meters) • Thyroid functions • Secondary sexual characteristics
2	Breasts	• Development • Related pathology • Occult galactorrhea
3	Chest	• Respiration • Circulatory system
4	Abdominal	• Discoloration of the skin (striae) • Surgical scars • Mass • Enlarged organ • Fluid in the abdomen (ascites)
5	Genital	• External examination • Per vaginal examination • Per speculum examination

Adopted from Kamel R: Management of the infertile couple: an evidence-based protocol, Reprod Biol Endocrinol 8(1):21, 2010. https://doi.org/10.1186/1477-7827-8-21.

Table 13.4 Infertility management protocol: general physical examination of male partner.

S. no.	Examination	Inclusions
1	General	• Blood pressure • Body height and weight (BMI) = ratio of weight (kilograms) with height (square meters) • Arm span assessment • Secondary sexual characteristics • Thyroid gland function
2	Breasts	• Gynecomastia
3	Abdominal	• Discoloration of the skin (striae) • Surgical scars • Mass in lower abdomen • Undescended testis • Fluid in the abdomen (ascites)
4	Genital	• Examination of external genitals • Testis • Epididymis and vas deferens • Per rectal (PR) examination for prostate enlargement

Adopted from Kamel R: Management of the infertile couple: an evidence-based protocol, Reprod Biol Endocrinol 8(1):21, 2010. https://doi.org/10.1186/1477-7827-8-21.

Table 13.5 Investigation protocols of a male partner with 12 months of infertility.

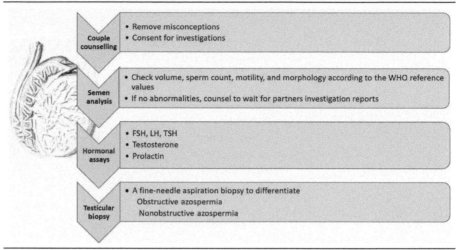

Couple counselling	• Remove misconceptions • Consent for investigations
Semen analysis	• Check volume, sperm count, motility, and morphology according to the WHO reference values • If no abnormalities, counsel to wait for partners investigation reports
Hormonal assays	• FSH, LH, TSH • Testosterone • Prolactin

Testicular biopsy	• A fine-needle aspiration biopsy to differentiate
	   Obstructive azospermia
	   Nonobstructive azospermia

Table 13.6 Investigation protocols of a female partner with 12 months of infertility.

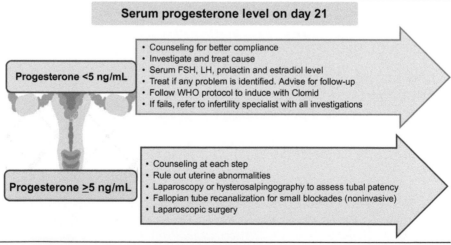

Serum progesterone level on day 21

Progesterone <5 ng/mL
• Counseling for better compliance
• Investigate and treat cause
• Serum FSH, LH, prolactin and estradiol level
• Treat if any problem is identified. Advise for follow-up
• Follow WHO protocol to induce with Clomid
• If fails, refer to infertility specialist with all investigations

Progesterone ≥5 ng/mL
• Counseling at each step
• Rule out uterine abnormalities
• Laparoscopy or hysterosalpingography to assess tubal patency
• Fallopian tube recanalization for small blockades (noninvasive)
• Laparoscopic surgery

https://www.ncbi.nlm.nih.gov/pmc/articles/PMC4609318

- Occupation: *Appropriate advice* should be offered.
- Couples should be told to *avoid over-the-counter and recreational drugs.*[2]
- Alcohol: *Both partners* should be informed about the *hazards of alcohol intake,* and "women who are trying to become pregnant should be informed that drinking no more than 1 or 2 units of alcohol once or twice per week and avoiding episodes of intoxication reduce the risk of harming a developing fetus." *"Men should be informed that excessive alcohol intake is detrimental to semen quality"* (Fig. 13.2).[2]

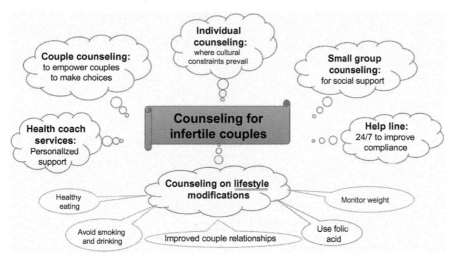

FIG. 13.2

Counseling of infertile couples.

Resolution to infertility

Resolution to infertility may or may not be a successful pregnancy. Finding resolution to infertility is the decision followed by a list of goals, options, plans, and strategies a couple selects for himself and his life partner. This is a difficult choice and a long journey that needs emotional and psychological support from friends, family, and the infertility specialists/counselors. A decision of adoption or to live childfree is yet another important resolution that has to be thought and discussed by the couple a number of times before putting into process.[23]

References

1. Ali S, Sophie R, Imam AM, et al. Knowledge, perceptions and myths regarding infertility among selected adult population in Pakistan: a cross-sectional study. *BMC Public Health.* 2011;11(1), 760.
2. Women's NCCf, Health Cs. *Fertility: Assessment and Treatment for People With Fertility Problems.* RCOG Press; 2004.
3. Burnett JA. Cultural considerations in counseling couples who experience infertility. *J Multicult Couns Dev.* 2009;37(3):166–177.
4. Yazdani F, Elyasi F, Peyvandi S, et al. Counseling-supportive interventions to decrease infertile women's perceived stress: a systematic review. *Electron Physician.* 2017;9(6):4694.
5. Pedro J, Brandão T, Schmidt L, Costa ME, Martins MV. What do people know about fertility? A systematic review on fertility awareness and its associated factors. *Ups J Med Sci.* 2018;123(2):71–81.

6. Adageba R, Maya E, Annan J, Damalie F. Setting up and running a successful IVF program in Africa: prospects and challenges. *J Obstet Gynaecol India.* 2015;65(3):155–157.

7. Wiltshire A, Brayboy LM, Phillips K, Matthews R, Yan F, McCarthy-Keith D. Infertility knowledge and treatment beliefs among African American women in an urban community. *Contracep Reprod Med.* 2019;4(1), 16.

8. Human Fertilisation and Embryology Authority Human Fertilisation and Embryology Authority Sixth Annual Report, 1997. 1997.

9. Klock SC. Psychosocial evaluation of the infertile patient. In: Covington SN, Burns LH, eds. *Infertility Counseling: A Comprehensive Handbook for Clinicians.* Cambridge University Press; 2006:83–96.

10. Jafarzadeh KF, Ghahiri A, Zargham BA, Habibi M. Exploration of the counseling needs of infertile couples: a qualitative study. *Iran J Nurs Midwifery Res.* 2015;20(5):552–559.

11. Vayena E, Rowe PJ, Griffin PD. *Current Practices and Controversies in Assisted Reproduction: Report of a Meeting on Medical, Ethical and Social Aspects of Assisted Reproduction, held at WHO Headquarters in Geneva, Switzerland.* World Health Organization; 2002.

12. Patel A, Sharma P, Kumar P. Role of mental health practitioner in infertility clinics: a review on past, present and future directions. *J Hum Reprod Sci.* 2018;11(3):219.

13. Van den Broeck U, Emery M, Wischmann T, Thorn P. Counselling in infertility: individual, couple and group interventions. *Patient Educ Couns.* 2010;81(3):422–428.

14. Bartlam B, McLeod J. Infertility counselling: the ISSUE experience of setting up a telephone counselling service. *Patient Educ Couns.* 2000;41(3):313–321.

15. Nekavand M, Mobini N, Roshandel S, Sheikhi A. A survey on the impact of relaxation on anxiety and the result of IVF in patients with infertility that have been referred to the infertility centers of Tehran university of medical sciences during 2012–2013. *Nurs Midwifery J.* 2015;13(7):605–612.

16. Valiani M, Abedian S, Ahmadi SM, Pahlavanzade S. The effects of relaxation on outcome treatment in infertile women. *Complement Med J Fac Nurs Midwifery.* 2014;4(2):845–853.

17. Kamel RM. Management of the infertile couple: an evidence-based protocol. *Reprod Biol Endocrinol.* 2010;8(1), 21.

18. Moura-Ramos M, Gameiro S, Canavarro MC, Soares I, Almeida-Santos TJ. Does infertility history affect the emotional adjustment of couples undergoing assisted reproduction? The mediating role of the importance of parenthood. *Br J Health Psychol.* 2016;21(2):302–317.

19. Rehman R, Zahid N, Amjad S, Baig M, Gazzaz ZJ. Relationship between smoking habit and sperm parameters among patients attending an infertility clinic. *Front Physiol.* 2019;10:1356.

20. Hart K, Tadros NN. The role of environmental factors and lifestyle on male reproductive health, the epigenome, and resulting offspring. *Iran J Nurs Midwifery Res.* 2019;61(2):187–195.

21. Collins GG, Rossi BV. The impact of lifestyle modifications, diet, and vitamin supplementation on natural fertility. *Fertil Res Pract.* 2015;1(1):11.

22. Rehman R, Hussain Z, Fatima SS. Effect of weight status on pregnancy outcome in intra cytoplasmic sperm injection. *Iran J Reprod Med.* 2013;11(9):717.

23. Siddiqui A, Desai NG, Sharma SB, Aslam M, Sinha UK, Madhu SV. Association of oxidative stress and inflammatory markers with chronic stress in patients with newly diagnosed type 2 diabetes. *Diabetes Metab Res Rev.* 2019;35(5), e3147.

Index

Note: Page numbers followed by *f* indicate figures and *t* indicate tables.